# Marriage Across Frontiers

# MULTILINGUAL MATTERS

Afrikaner Dissidents
  JOHA LOUW-POTGIETER
Aspects of Bilingualism in Wales
  COLIN BAKER
Australian Multiculturalism
  LOIS FOSTER and DAVID STOCKLEY
Bilingual Children: From Birth to Teens
  GEORGE SAUNDERS
Bilingualism or Not: The Education of Minorities
  TOVE SKUTNABB-KANGAS
Bilingualism: Basic Principles
  HUGO BAETENS BEARDSMORE
Communication and Cross-cultural Adaptation
  YOUNG YUN KIM
Cultural Studies in Foreign Language Education
  MICHAEL BYRAM
English in Wales: Diversity, Conflict and Change
  NIKOLAS COUPLAND (ed.)
Evaluating Bilingual Education
  MERRILL SWAIN and SHARON LAPKIN
The Interdisciplinary Study of Urban Bilingualism in Brussels
  E. WITTE and H. BAETENS BEARDSMORE (eds.)
Key Issues in Bilingualism and Bilingual Education
  COLIN BAKER
Language Acquisition of a Bilingual Child
  ALVINO FANTINI
Language Attitudes Among Arabic-French Bilinguals in Morocco
  ABDELÂLI BENTAHILA
Language and Ethnicity in Minority Sociolinguistic Perspective
  JOSHUA FISHMAN
Language in a Black Community
  VIV EDWARDS
Minority Education: From Shame to Struggle
  T. SKUTNABB-KANGAS and J. CUMMINS (eds.)
Minority Education and Ethnic Survival
  MICHAEL BYRAM
The Moving Experience
  GAIL MELTZER and ELAINE GRANDJEAN
Multiculturalism: The Changing Australian Paradigm
  LOIS FOSTER and DAVID STOCKLEY
Oral Language Across the Curriculum
  DAVID CORSON
Perspectives on Marital Interaction
  P. NOLLER and M.A. FITZPATRICK (eds.)
Pluralism: Cultural Maintenance and Evolution
  BRIAN BULLIVANT
Raising Children Bilingually: The Pre-School Years
  LENORE ARNBERG
Young Children in China
  R. LILJESTRÖM et al.

**Please contact us for the latest book information:**
**Multilingual Matters,**
**Bank House, 8a Hill Rd, Clevedon, Avon BS21 7HH, England.**

# Marriage Across Frontiers

Augustin Barbara

Translated by David E. Kennard

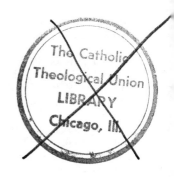

**MULTILINGUAL MATTERS LTD**
Clevedon · Philadelphia

**Library of Congress Cataloging in Publication Data**
Barbara, Augustin.
  Marriage across frontiers.
  Translation of: Mariages sans Frontières.
  Bibliography: p.
  1. Intermarriage.  2. Interracial marriage.
I. Title.
HQ1031.B33613  1989  306.8′43  88-34538


**British Library Cataloguing in Publication Data**
Barbara, Augustin
  Marriage across frontiers.
  1. Marriage
  I. Title  II. Mariages sans Frontières.
  *English*
  306.8′1

  ISBN 1-85359-042-8
  ISBN 1-85359-041-X pbk


**Multilingual Matters Ltd**
Bank House, 8a Hill Road      &      242 Cherry Street
Clevedon, Avon BS21 7HH              Philadelphia, Pa 19106–1906
England                              U.S.A.

Copyright © 1989  Augustin Barbara
Translated by David E. Kennard

First published 1985 under the
title 'Mariages Sans Frontières'
by Bayarde Press, S.A., 'Editions
du Centurion, Paris', France.

Cover design by Busen
Typeset by Editorial Enterprises, Torquay, Devon
Printed and bound in Great Britain by WBC Print Ltd, Bristol

# Contents

## PART 4: HOPES AND REALITIES

# Preface

The main question to be asked by every human being is 'who am I?'; one of the ways to begin to answer this question is to pose another question: 'Who made me?'. Every man, Jean-Paul Sartre tells us, is 'made by all men'. But in this creation of one person by all the others, some people have a privileged role to play.

The geneticist's attention is focused primarily on the two procreators: the meeting of the ovum and the sperm brings into being all those biological ingredients with which the organism will be able to develop little by little, resisting the attacks of the outside world, acquiring innumerable powers according to the rhythm of its own internal clock until it finally collapses and is absorbed. But all these contributions are the basic 'bricks' with which the whole is built; by confining our questions to the characteristics of these elements, we are able to approach the essential part: the architecture of their arrangement. The important thing is the progressive structuring which makes a person of each human being.

Depending on the culture, this structuring is brought about primarily by the couple who conceived the child, by close or distant relatives, by siblings, or by friends of the same age ... But their contributions are limited in the main to childhood and adolescence, since each of us has the whole of life in which to become, day by day, what we choose to be.

In our cultures, where the stated ideal is the stability of the couple, those who come together as a couple are participating not only in the creation of their children, but just as certainly in their own self-realisation. The things we are enthusiastic and excited about, shared intimacies, as well as the difficulties, knocks and conflicts, have a transforming effect on both partners as they interact.

The dynamics thus created are even more powerful, and the risks greater, when the distance between the two people concerned is a marked one. The first dimension of this distance is that they belong to the two 'races' into which people are divided: female and male. However, other dimensions can add to this distance: culture, religion, philosophical outlook and politics.

Our culture has invented a term to describe couples in which one or several of these additional distances is present: 'mixed marriages' (as though all marriages were not 'mixed'!). It is to this study of mixed marriages that Augustin Barbara has devoted many years of research.

At a first reading the information he gives us and the thoughts he develops enable us to better understand the extent of this leprosy in our society: contempt which is justified by the fact of belonging to a certain group, in other words racism. The make-up of a couple can be a catalyst for exposing the most camouflaged and the most unconscious racist feelings; the presence of a 'mixed' couple is a major scandal for those who are unable to see any truth apart from their own. A thousand and one tricks are employed and destructive forces are unleashed in order to spoil things, ending with the deadly pronouncement: 'I told you so'.

But Augustin Barbara's analysis does not stop there; it also sheds light on the dynamics of all couples. So-called mixed couples serve as a useful example, they are like a laboratory experiment in which conditions of extreme tension are created, thereby revealing the mechanisms at work in milder cases. It has to do with being confronted with another person, existing in that person's presence, but it also has to do with being transformed by the other person; the result is a so-called life 'in common', but in such a way that each person is able to find, in this community, the source of his or her own personal adventure. The laws governing this mysterious and paradoxical alchemy are all the more readily discernible when the constraints in operation are severe and when the obstacles put up by those around are many in number. The paths trod by couples in which one partner is French and the other N.W. African, or in which one partner is Muslim and the other Christian (or Franco-American, Franco-German, Judeo-Christian, or even couples in which one partner is from the French West Indies and the other is from the motherland, etc.) are therefore revealing adventures, and the lessons to be drawn from them can be valuable for couples that are somewhat less mixed, for example where both partners are French or where both partners are Muslim, etc.

Our consideration of the personal development of each human being in the context of other people and thanks to those other people is engaged by Augustin Barbara with respect to the specific example of the couple in which people are in a one-to-one relationship.

Albert Jacquard
*Geneticist*
*National Institute of Demographic Studies, Paris*

# 1 Introduction

The idea of writing a book on mixed marriages became firmly implanted in my mind as the result of a conversation on a train. When my fellow traveller heard that I was engaged in research on marriage, she confided that her brother was married to a West Indian and that she herself had lived for several years with a Japanese man. She paused for some time before deciding to add:

A Westerner will come right to the point in a conversation, whereas a Japanese takes an entirely different approach. You get the impression that he is almost trying to avoid a subject before finally tackling it. He must have time. And this wasn't easy for me because I always like things to be clear from the start; whereas he felt a need for things to become clear bit by bit. (. . .) We lived together for several years, and though there were lots of areas in which we saw eye to eye, I always found talking to him very difficult. By the end my Japanese was getting better and better. I began to understand his different way of seeing things. But would I always be able to accept it? That's what worried me.

She went on to tell me how discovering the Zen monastery garden of Ryoanji near Kyoto had amazed her and unsettled her by its simplicity. The masterly positioning of fifteen stones on a sea of sand leads the visitor into a space which is purposefully laid out not only for the eyes but for the whole body. It is a sort of all-embracing microclimate in which smells, colours and even differences in temperature between one corner of the garden and another each play their part. One's whole body is caught up in a sensory experience.

I was quite sure that in a real sense they were very different from us. For instance, it irritated me never to take the same route to the same place. The streets of cities often don't have a name and the house numbers aren't in any logical order but follow their date of construction. I was always getting lost. I felt all right in Paris. He found it easier to adapt to France than I did to his country. In the end I was the one who didn't want to carry on.

She added that her family had played a significant part in this decision. 'The family is more tolerant of a man who marries a foreigner than of a woman who marries a foreigner.'

Her parents' reactions were different towards her brother and his West Indian wife. They simply refused to take it seriously. 'It won't last long', they thought. To begin with they were basically against this marriage, because of the colour of the young woman's skin. 'She's not the right sort of girl for him.' But as time passed, they came to accept her, particularly after they had a child!

It was the less favourable reactions of her family to her own situation which caused her to reject the idea of marrying her Japanese partner whom she loved very much. 'Yes, my family was really more tolerant in my brother's case.'

A four-hour train journey gives you the opportunity to get to know people and the life they lead. She informed me that she had recently married a Frenchman who had been posted to Curacao. He had come 'to choose her' on that Dutch island in the West Indies where she was the only French woman. She was teaching French there. 'Only mountains keep themselves to themselves', she said.

Her experience and marriage caused me to think seriously of the complexity of mixed marriages and at the same time about the complexity of a certain type of logic. What determines the lasting nature of a relationship when two individuals come together is the relative resistance of the groups to which they belong. Is it not the case that a so-called 'good match' between a Frenchman posted to a Caribbean island and the only French woman on the island is itself a mixed marriage from certain points of view? He comes from Brittany, she is from Lorraine; there would be little likelihood of their having met one another in France. It would seem in this case that chance has acted in response to unforeseeable circumstances. What if this same Frenchman working abroad had met another solitary French woman on a neighbouring island! . . .

***

It is a warm afternoon in July and a mixed couple is strolling along the street in Chinatown, New York. There are obvious signs of affection between them and they talk freely as they stand in front of a shop window that displays Chinese goods. This is a picture of the United States.

Everyday life in America has its moments of utmost humanity in the shadow of the Empire State Building or Wall Street. But many prejudices had to be overcome before a black man and a white woman could walk openly together in New York without raising a few eyebrows. Can we really say that there are many couples like this and that they are perfectly accepted? No, proportionally they represent a small percentage of marriages. The anonymous environment of the American city is the perfect place for looking like everyone else, which often means not being noticed! In some of the Southern states, on the other hand, mixed couples stand out and are strongly disapproved of. They do not have the benefit of the undisturbed freedom or the right to go unnoticed. No one points to a mixed couple in the Place de la Concorde in Paris. It is the side streets of the suburbs, in a small provincial town well off the beaten track that people will make a point of mentioning the fact that 'so-and-so is going out with a black man or an Arab.'

However, among the coloured children playing near the Golden Triangle in Pittsburgh (Pennsylvania), where the Monongahela, the Alleghany and the Ohio flow together, a number of them have physical characteristics of a slightly Negroid or Hispanic type, along with blue eyes, a mat complexion and light brown hair. These children play together under a jet of water in the setting sun, unaware that they are the living synthesis of a series of human wanderings which goes back many generations. 'Crossbreeding is one of the basic principles of life', writes Professor Jacques Ruffié.[1]

Crossbreeding is a prerequisite for the proper functioning of society. To quote Jacques Ruffié again: 'A pure race is always a fragile race, with no long-term future. Genetic polymorphism represents the norm for the species.'[2]

It seems then that we are nothing more than the product of crossbreeding way back in time. Any groups which clung to their isolation in time and space would not have survived! Is mixed marriage necessary? The geneticist has no qualms about this:

> Speaking as a geneticist, I've come to the point where I can no longer define a mixed marriage, because marriage in our society is by nature mixed in that the two individuals involved are different in their own ways. One of them is male and the other female. That is where the true mix and the true distance lie.[3]

One cannot help admitting therefore that genes are more readily able to cross racial barriers than cultural ones. The work carried out by

Professor Jacques Ruffié on the Cape Verde islands, some 280 miles from Dakar, whose total area is equivalent to that of half of Corsica, is interesting in this respect. The strategic position they occupy on the route to Brazil did not escape the attention of the first Portuguese colonists who discovered these islands in 1460, taking up residence there from 1462 onwards. Thereafter the islands served as a depot for African slaves in the triangular trade between Europe, Africa and the new continent. The Portuguese mixed with some of the imported black slaves and brought into being a population (272,000 inhabitants in 1976) that is so thoroughly mixed that to be all black or all white is now considered as 'abnormal'. Moreover, there are not really any physical, territorial boundaries separating the Whites and the Blacks in this world. In one and the same area one passes from black to white in a continuous series of variations, in successive degrees.

'A marriage will be mixed, from the racial point of view, according to where one chooses to draw the dividing line. And where one draws this line is completely arbitrary.'[4] This is the case in the South Africa of the Afrikaners.

There is of course, and we all learned it back in our schooldays, an ideology which sees mankind as divided up into colours. This ideology separates, distinguishes, distributes men and women into different races. This way of looking at things has been developed to its logical extreme of institutionalising the difference in the form of inequality. From early childhood, depending on the environment and country in which we grow up, this difference is institutionalised to a greater or lesser degree in our thinking in the form of a functional inequality which 'segregates' and separates White from Black, establishing a whole hierarchy of shades, religions, values, languages, etc. It is something we inherit. It is a sort of poisoned gift, like a heavy load which we must carry around and which we are unable to get rid of. Reality seems quite different. Can it be simple when the phenomenon itself seems so complex? However clear-cut it may appear for genetics, it is an infinitely complex matter for human sciences.

* * *

Nevertheless mixed marriage, or intercultural marriage would seem to be a fairly accurate indicator of the progress in a society which is involved in integration, assimilation and the mixing of individuals in order that conflicts and competition might be avoided. It is also an indicator of the nature of that society's identity. Is it moving towards loss and fragmentation, or is it moving towards a transformation which will be of benefit for all its members? All peoples and all groups have to face this question. The whole of human history consists of such questions.

As long as mankind has existed, groups of people have perceived the need to live together. Whether at war or at peace, these contacts have always resulted in marriages outside of the group. Well defined and controlled or not, it was the group which determined the rules on marriage, aimed at ensuring its geographic, economic and demographic survival. No group ever cheerfully allows itself to die out. History shows us that quite the opposite is the case! How many threatened, decimated or exterminated groups there have been which have fought tooth and nail to spring back to life so as to regain importance and a place among other groups! But marriage with an outsider, too, can become dangerous if it is widespread. One only has to look at how Athens regulated marriage for its citizens so that only a certain number of mixed marriages were permitted, often ruling them out altogether. During the exodus of the Jewish people, such marriages were forbidden because they weakened the physical potential of the group at the very time when it needed every ounce of strength it had. It is a continuous theme throughout history.

This type of marriage has always raised a number of questions at a general and social level, even though at first glance it would seem to be nothing more than an intimate matter between two individuals who love one another. Now the weaker a society or group is, the stricter, and sometimes more constraining, will be the rules governing marriage for women. Every social group, in keeping a close watch on how its members choose their marriage partners, wants to guarantee its survival and not allow itself to be swallowed up, particularly by not allowing its women to go outside of the group. This surely is what has happened in some rural districts of France where the exodus of women led in a few years to the depopulation of mountainous areas? The celibate peasants, growing old alongside their aged parents, continued their activities for a few years in order to survive, but there were no children to hand their livelihoods down to. Of course, it was not without good reason that the young women left . . .

This question is still a relevant one and in Georges Friedman's book *Fin du Peuple Juif* [The End of the Jewish People] it is at the centre of the upsurge of the international Jewish community. Must it allow itself to be assimilated into all the peoples, nations and countries to which it has been scattered? 'For this people, which has lived almost two thousand years without territory of its own, struggling against persecution or threatened by assimilation and oblivion in, the host communities, the founding of a home remains essential.[5] In some countries maintaining a Jewish identity precluded the complete merger with another people, and helped to maintain a minimum level of marriages between Jews. The Armenian people, annihilated by the genocide of 1915, was able to survive thanks to a minimum number of men and women below which no conscious sense of community can exist.

There are many countries which still have restrictive regulations on mixed marriages, so much so that the agreements from the Helsinki Conference of August 1975 devoted one of its chapters to the private movement of persons. The last Conference in Madrid, July 1983, was more explicit. The final document states the new provisions on the reunion of families and goes one step further than those drawn up at the Helsinki Conference: 'Participating states will grant favourable treatment to the requests which have to do with contact and regular meetings on the basis of family ties, with the reuniting of families and with marriages between citizens of different states, and will respond to such requests in the same spirit.' A meeting of experts was held in Ottawa on 7th May 1985 with a view to drawing up even clearer conclusions and guidelines.[6]

There are, indeed, numerous cases of fiancés or married couples separated by physical or legal barriers. Not a year goes by without Franco-Rumanian husbands or wives staging a hunger strike in order to be reunited with their partners. The marriage between the French woman Odile Pierquin and the Chinese Ti Han Li was only able to take place through the mediation of the top people in each country. Mr Bellefroid, the diplomat, was considered to be *persona non grata* by the popular Chinese authorities and his fiancée, Li-Shuang, was sent to a re-education camp. This romance led to a diplomatic incident during a visit by a French minister of state, Mr Michel Jobert, in November 1981. Li-Shuang, an artist, was allowed to join her fiancé in Paris in July 1983.[7] They were married on 4th February 1984. In contrast, after only six months waiting, another Chinese artist, the sculptor Wang Keping married a French woman working in China, Miss Catherine Dezaly, on 30th December 1981 in Peking.[8] In South Africa mixed marriage was, until recently, forbidden and punishable by imprisonment, as was any sexual contact with coloured partners.

Thus we can see that within groups, nations and states there are differing levels of response to such marriages taking place. At the same time, there are a number of factors which encourage such unions. One only has to spend an afternoon at Orly or Roissy to realise how mobile people are in the twentieth century. Thousands of people arrive from all countries of the world. They had only just left them a short while before. Holiday migrations, stays or study periods abroad, the exchange of personnel and the considerable immigration of workers into countries where there is the offer of employment are some of the phenomena which cause millions of men and women to move around. The development of international bodies, congresses, conferences and gatherings of all sorts (scientific, commercial, sports), all contribute towards moving individuals from one place to another for varying lengths of time. On top of this are the unhappy forced and painful migrations we see in the countless refugees of present day wars. They leave their homes by road, boat and plane, and become separated in their host countries. We could even say that the growing trend of adopting foreign children is itself a form of migration.

In each case individuals forming a minority group are placed for a certain length of time in the midst of an indigenous majority population. They stay there for a certain period of time, leave or settle for good in a new place. Whether it be temporary or permanent (or permanently temporary), their stay gives them ample opportunity to form links with the host population. Some of them will go so far as to marry natives of that country, thereby showing an even greater willingness to settle down in the country.

*\*\**

The number of mixed marriages is becoming increasingly significant. To take France as an example, there was a rise of 1.5% in just seven years: 6.5% in 1981, compared with 5% in 1974. In the period between 1975 and 1981 there were a total of 143,321 mixed marriages out of a total number of 2,473,400 marriages, that is to say around 5.80% of marriages, whereas in the earlier period of 1968 to 1974 there were 130,550 mixed marriages out of a total of 2,749,652, that is to say 4.75%[9]. One fact emerges from this: although the overall number of marriages is decreasing in French society, the number of mixed marriages seems to be steady at just over 20,000 a year (20,319 in 1981, but 30,480 in 1946 at the end of the Second World War!). These figures do not reflect the marriage figures for French people overseas with partners from the mother country which can, from some points of view, be considered as intercultural marriages, even if they do not involve two nationalities. Nor is it possible to count the number of mixed partners cohabiting.

On the one hand, choice, constraint and the need to move, in general terms, have consequences for the lives of individuals, because these things to some extent upset the general rules by which societies operate. On the other hand, at the level of people's personal lives, these consequences affect individuals at the heart of their intimate lives, and for a long period of time. How can two people who are completely alien to one another take such a great risk, undertaking to live together in this experience which requires a great understanding of one another? Incomprehension is built in right at the start of their relationship and how will they manage to deal with a whole host of situations, problems and conflicts? And if not incomprehension, is it enough to be willing to understand and accept one's partner? Is this willingness alone enough for one to be able to express one's differences without reserve?

## The Mixed Couple: A Typical Example of the Union Between Two Individuals

Mixed (or intercultural) marriage — we will come back to these terms later — is often portrayed as a separate type of marriage, or it at least attracts attention. It is seen as a stretching of the normal rules governing the formation of marriages. For this reason, this type of marriage can serve as an example to help us at various levels of our understanding.

MIXED MARRIAGES IN FRANCE (1975–1981)

| Year | Partners | | | | |
|------|----------|---|---|---|---|
| | French man foreign woman | French woman foreign man | Total of mixed marriages | Total marriages (000s) | Percentage of mixed marriages |
| 1975 | 7,918 | 12,698 | 20,616 | 387.4 | 5.3% |
| 1976 | 7,677 | 12,481 | 20,158 | 374.0 | 5.4% |
| 1977 | 7,940 | 12,839 | 20,779 | 368.0 | 5.6% |
| 1978 | 7,957 | 12,608 | 20,565 | 354.6 | 5.8% |
| 1979 | 7,938 | 12,332 | 20,270 | 340.4 | 6.0% |
| 1980 | 8,323 | 12,292 | 20,615 | 334.4 | 6.2% |
| 1981 | 8,257 | 12,061 | 20,318 | 314.6(p) | 6.5% |
| TOTALS | 56,010 | 87,311 | 143,321 | 2,473.4 | |
| PERCENT-AGE | 39.1 | 60.9 | 100 | 100 | 5.8 |

p = estimate                                         (Source: INSEE, civil records)

MIXED MARRIAGES (COMPARISON BETWEEN TWO PERIODS)

| | *Marriages* | | |
|---|---|---|---|
| *Periods* | *Total of marriages* | *Mixed marriages* | *Percentage* |
| A. 1968–1974 | 2,749,562 | 130,550 | 4.75% |
| B. 1975–1981 | 2,473,400 | 143,321 | 5.80% |
| Difference A/B | -276,162 | +12,771 | +1.05% |

(Source: INSEE, civil records)

The recurring theme throughout this book is simple. It can be read from two different perspectives. On the one hand mixed marriage enables us to understand the social logic that is behind all unions of individuals. Marriage is in effect a universal social fact, but it takes different forms according to the societies, cultures and religions within which it takes place. Mixed marriage highlights certain mechanisms which , even if they are a factor of those special circumstances, nevertheless allow us to make certain generalisations. On the other hand, at a much more micro-psycho-sociological level, it very quickly demonstrates situations which couples have to go through, for the reason that at certain times couples are unable to express the truth of a marriage relationship because of certain irreducible distances.

The dual level on which this book is written therefore enables us to reflect on marriage in general and on the couple in particular, starting out from examples and specific situations lived out by mixed couples. On the basis of university research.[10] I have chosen to adopt a form of writing which was geared at one and the same time to readers who were familiar with intercultural relations and readers familiar with the transforming effect being part of a couple has on life. Both cultural interaction and the life of couples are currently in a state of change. Cultural interaction is an historic fact: because of the new technological conditions of existence, people can no longer remain in isolation. Exchanges of all sorts — economic, commercial, cultural, sports, political and university, etc. — are taking place at an ever faster rate. It is no longer possible to ignore one's neighbour on the other side of the world. As for the couple — that union of two people — never before has it been so discussed and questioned as though, for the first time, the enormous potential benefits it conceals had suddenly been discovered as it undergoes different stages of development:

the challenging confrontation of two free entities in lasting relationships of intensity of loving sentiment.

Another concern guided me in writing this book: that of the place and the status of children in these new areas of difficulty. After all, are not children also the centre of what is at stake in any union — be it lasting or transitory — between a man and a woman? The importance of this aspect of the subject has grown considerably with the dramatic questions, or questions which tend to be dramatised in western societies at least, relating on the one hand to the drop in the birth rate and the desire to have children, and on the other hand to the current 'boom' in the area of divorce.

What this book is providing readers with is a reading of these facts through the illumination that can be gleaned from this type of marriage which is 'unlike the others'.


**Notes to Chapter 1**

1. De la biologie à la culture. From *Biology to Culture*, Paris: Flammarion, 1976, p. 103.
2. Ibid.
3. Albert Jacquard, Head of the Genetics of Populations department at INED (the National Institute of Demographic Studies), extracts from Dialogue de France-Culture with Augustin Barbara: 'Les mariages mixtes' [Mixed marriages], 11th July 1978; broadcast produced by Roger Pillaudin, Radio-France.
4. Ibid.
5. Luc Rosenzweig, 'Mariages difficiles dans la communauté juive' [Difficult marriages in the Jewish Community], *Le Monde Dimanche*, 30th November 1980.
6. *Le Monde*, 8th September 1983.
7. *Le Monde*, 11th November 1981.
8. *Le Monde*, 6th January 1982.
9. INSEE, civil records.
10. A. Barbara, 'Mariages mixtes' [Mixed marriages]. Thesis presented at the EHESS (the College for Higher Studies in Social Sciences), 400 pp., Paris, 1978.

# Part 1
# The Encounter

# 2 The choice of the other

*'O, strange partner ...'*

'Why did she want to marry that black man? She wasn't stuck for choice. There are plenty of young men around here!' Indeed, why and when does a member of a given community marry a foreigner? And, indeed, why not?

All these questions are raised in families whenever a young woman or man marries in a way which does not please those close to them. After all, they had always had in mind such-and-such a potential partner from among their acquaintances who would have been very suitable. And suddenly this strange partner arrives from far away! Everyone is very curious in anticipation of the first meeting when they can 'examine' this stranger. The group then lets its imagination run away with itself: 'Just think, with a name like that ... And what if they have children, has she thought about that? When they grow up with frizzy hair and large lips ...' It is the expression of their spontaneous, unrestrained fear of this *other* person who has never been seen in the village before.

Yet a few decades ago this same fear was being expressed, perhaps with less intensity, when the new partner came from a neighbouring village. The majority of marriages have always come into being within a limited geographic range. Before France was a national entity, each region or province regarded its neighbour as foreign, if not as a rival. The large towns were in competition with one another and the marriages which brought their inhabitants together were concluded with this in mind. In the eighteenth century anyone not born in the village of Dole was considered to be a foreigner. And those outsiders in the town married among themselves with partners from outside. In this small town in the French Jura the very watertight social compartments encouraged marriages between partners of the same social class whilst excluding outsiders. What a difficult time was experienced by an engaged couple, both of them Christian, who were separated because one was Catholic and the other Protestant! If these obstacles no longer exist in France, they remain just as prevalent in certain other countries.

'Moreover, if she found a partner from outside, it must be because of some special reason'. One young woman waited too long, another was too demanding and refused a succession of interested parties! 'The longer she waited, the harder it became for her; in the end she had to make do with a foreigner'. This popular notion sometimes expresses, with a naive force, the sort of thinking which goes on when two individuals meet. Why then do they not marry as the majority of people do and seem unhappy to choose partners in accordance with the accepted rules? Is it not the case that these well tried rules will lead more certainly and more easily to lasting happiness?

Despite all these assurances, the individuals in question nevertheless take on additional risks. Their union becomes an adventure. An adventure which is enticing just because of the unknown element it may contain.

I knew all the girls in my neighbourhood, the girls I had gone out with. I knew their families, the story of their lives. We had been baptised, confirmed and gone to school together. We were already engaged in a cycle of similar activities and in the end, if I had married one of them, I would have felt that there was nothing to discover. For me, marriage meant something to discover and not just the end of something. My idea was that I wanted to have to discover a person and, with that person, a whole new country, to discover something new. Yes, I look on marriage as a somewhat risky adventure, and that's what attracted me to my wife who is a foreigner. The other women were too familiar for one of them to become my wife (Frenchman, aged 30).

A desire to escape for this man who thus rationalises his choice of a foreign woman as an attempt to get away from his original group. We are right at the heart of romanticism here. But he chose a lifestyle abroad which takes him further and further away from his origins. His integration into his wife's society is stressed by his conversion to Islam and by the way in which his children are being brought up as Muslims. Ill at ease, or feeling himself to be an outsider, in his environment, he opted for another. He was converted and naturalised to a considerable extent. He has thereby abandoned everything which might reunite him to his original group. He has formed bonds elsewhere, perhaps because the first ones were not strong enough or because they were too oppressive (maybe he wanted to run away from them or break them). His marriage could be the sign of a crisis of independence from his relatives. The sudden desire for something new, in itself, would not explain this escape. Indeed, how is one to understand this strange desire, if not as the conscious or unconscious yearning for an element of risk?

In some U.S. states of the South a black man often ran the risk of being lynched if he wanted to 'go out with a white woman' not that many years ago. All sexual relations between partners of different colours were, until recently, forbidden in South Africa. Indeed, is it not the case that to marry outside of one's race and original group is also to violate the sexual taboo which is one of the strongest for a group's identity? G. Conchon's novel *L'État Sauvage*[1] [The Wild State] sheds light on the way in which the two groups, African and European, live side by side, each 'wildly' maintaining its own identity. Each side despises any individual who has chosen to live in a different way and uses degrading terms to describe that person.

This encounter between two different persons involves the simultaneous effects of attraction and fear. In G. Conchon's book we see a European who is obsessed by the fear of a black African getting too close to the white woman, while at the same time he himself has a strong desire to 'go to bed' with a black woman. Black woman, white woman, it is the woman who becomes the forbidden person according to the social rules of each group. Once the first encounter has taken place it quickly becomes a secret which is only continued on certain conditions and in certain places well away from the eyes and comments of others.

I was with some friends on the beach and when it was time to leave I realised I'd lost my car-keys in the sand. They helped us to find them. Even though they'd been right next to us all day we hadn't noticed them because they were foreigners. Then I went out with one of them . . . and now here I am married to him . . . (French woman).

This meeting would seem to be attributable to chance. Yet that is not quite the case. On the one hand we have a group of men, foreign workers, spending one Sunday in summer on a beach far from their homeland. And on the other hand we have three young female workers, originally from the country, that is to say strangers to the town, who have also gone for a relaxing day on the nearest beach. Moreover, the resemblance between the ways in which they live, work and spend their leisure time might well have been decisive in fostering a continuation of their meeting one another, leading, as in this case, as far as marriage itself. It might have been different if the young woman had been a doctor's daughter who had been brought up in the town instead of a farmer's daughter who had been obliged to find work in the town. In the case of a doctor's daughter or someone from a higher social class, the development of this encounter with a foreigner, a black man for instance, could take the form of a challenge thrown out to her social group. She may have had a very strict upbringing and might therefore allow this encounter to develop as a form of unconscious revenge.

Many of these young women are not bad and they come from
well-to-do families; they've had a very strict upbringing without the
chance to spread their wings. They delight in going round with a black
man. What they are trying to say is: 'Well I . . . but it's your racism,
your ideas'. They are rebelling against a whole upbringing which they
have not properly digested (French official, aged 42).

They are putting on an act for their family group. At the same time
they are testing out relations with the whole of their social group. This
event will now bring to light certain rifts which no one has yet suspected.
Sympathies will crumble: 'Good heavens, I know it's her own business,
a friend said to me, but she might have shown some consideration for you
and the way you brought her up' (Frenchman, aged 48, whose daughter
married a man from Senegal). In order not to provoke comments which
can, at times, be very unpleasant, the lovers will conduct their relationship
with a certain amount of discretion which, by reinforcing their isolation,
will also consolidate their relationship and may even lead them into too
hasty a choice.

My family never dreamed I would marry a black African. I was a well
brought up girl, having more in common with a nun than the young
French girl who goes around flirting. I was very impressed when he
sat next to me in the Faculty lecture room. At last I was observing
a 'Negro' at close quarters. He was the first one to engage in
conversation. We got into the habit of sitting together. One day I
borrowed his course notes. His writing was not only good, it was
impeccable. And that together with very well spoken French. One day
I realised he was handsome. And I began to fantasise about him. I
destroyed within myself an old idea of the black man which had been
passed on to me by my family. It was then that a real attraction for
him began. On his side, his reserve only served to add to my
frustration. Suddenly I felt a desire to make love with him. And I can
assure you I was not disappointed. Yes, it was I, the timid girl, who
made the advances. For some months we lived out a secret dream. It
was great . . . He really made me feel I was a women . . . (French
student, aged 25).

The period of secrecy was followed by one of challenge. Now sure of
herself and valuing their relationship very much, she wanted to impose this
new situation on her family. Knowing that they would not understand
straight away, she opted for a sort of provocation:

Many of my friends left me; I found others who were able to accept
my black boyfriend. It was a great change of environment. In this new

situation I discovered a whole range of people I'd never had anything to do with before. And a great many preconceived ideas were wiped out at a stroke. My boyfriend, who was a stranger to this society, had been instrumental in enabling me to understand my own society better, at least a certain part of it (Idem).

This personal account highlights certain mechanisms of an encounter in which fascination for the other is bound up with a strong attraction. This more or less secret period in a relationship comes before a challenge which would seem to be the necessary transition to obtaining public recognition or social exclusion. We see it here in the form of the expression of opinions by friends, those who are sympathetic and those who are sceptical . . . and those who say to one another: 'Let's see how long it lasts . . .' The same people who, if the couple goes through a difficult patch, will say: 'I knew it, it was only a question of time . . . if only she'd listened to us in the first place . . .'

The sexual aspect of this encounter is important. Indeed a mixed couple can be the scene for a cultural confrontation between two individuals who have different sexual languages. Alongside these different languages which can be identified objectively there is also the whole realm of fantasy about the sexuality of the other. Moreover, the adventurous quest to know a forbidden desire increases this sexual preoccupation. The film *L'État Sauvage* [The Wild State] clearly portrays the conceit of the white man when the black man looks at the white woman. John Griffin in his book *In the Skin of a Black Man*[2] states this point of view very clearly: 'Even if you do not realise that you are looking in the direction of a white woman they will try to make something of it'. The white woman symbolises the feminine part of the common ego of white people. This means that she is no longer an isolated individual, but an integral part of a social group which, if it has any contact — especially of a sexual nature — with another group, will lose its integrity and its identity. To go to bed with a black man is perceived as an insult which strikes at the most intimate part of white people. Moreover, the supposed sexual power of the black man, which is at the back of the white man's mind, is a direct threat. The white man believes that the white woman sees the black man as having greater sexual prowess than the white man has. He feels not only threatened but also perhaps inadequate . . .

By the same token the white woman forms part of the mythical dream of the black man: half goddess, half woman. An opposition is established between a white world in which the attraction, beauty and purity of the woman is valued, and a black world with its primitive, wild sexuality. This blurring of concepts, this unknown territory increases the keen desire of going to bed with the other person. This fascination has very deep roots in the ideas going around, particularly with regard to the qualities or defects attributed to various nationalities or physical types according to sex. It is for this reason that the Swedish blonde fascinates the Mediterraneans and that Asian or Eurasian women have an over-whelmingly seductive effect on the French male!

> More and more men are travelling to Asia. They are drawn by the Asian woman. It's the image of her body, of the indigenous Indo-Chinese woman, that persists. Then there are the Thai massage parlours . . . It is nothing more than a search for a new type of sexuality ( . . .). After they've been once they go again the next year and come back with a wife. Some of them remain there. They look for a job with a multinational company . . . (An employee in a travel agency).

A whole hierarchy of attraction and fascination seems to be taking shape, although it is not always a conscious thing:

> It's quite clear-cut, for far-off countries where men are in the majority. As far as the Mediterranean countries are concerned, it is essentially women. We went on a trip to Greece: there were twice as many women as men (Idem).

If men travel further afield it is perhaps because they have more opportunity and because their professional positions mean that they earn more than women. Thus an encounter is not always the result of chance, it may be a response to expectations. Sometimes it is even a straight-forward result of a deliberate strategy, a calculated move:

> I didn't have a job. Now I'm on a scheme[3]. But if I don't find work at the end of this scheme, I could be sent back the day after. And I don't want to go back to Morocco, I have no family there. It was my uncle who took me in here, because my own family are all dead. The best solution if I am to stay in France would be for me to marry a French girl. Then, I think, I'd have a chance of staying in France . . . (Moroccan, aged 19, trainee).

This strategy encapsulates a number of different aspects. Determined by the personal circumstance of unemployment, the search for a job and the performance of that job are tied up with the related possibility of settling in France. Is it not the case that many mixed marriages have been due to successive waves of immigration since the beginning of the century? Thus, the choice of a foreign partner is not quite as free as the majority of mixed couples would like to think it is:

We had nothing in common. How else could you explain that if it weren't love. Scarcely three months ago he was still living in his own country. In this case it is really a combination of love and chance . . . (French student, aged 24, from a farming background).

The force of expression of this young woman student confirm the whole concept of love which tends to reinforce mixed marriages. She had only come to town in order to study, three days a week, never succeeding in making friends among her fellow students. She was the only daughter of a farmer; there seemed to be no place for her in this world of townspeople, especially among the students who were for the most part the children of higher social classes and who made her feel uncomfortable about her own background. Being in a sense an exile in an environment where she was not at ease, she found herself in a similar position to that of this foreign student who had come to study in the same town as her. He too had left his natural surroundings. The same department, the same lecture rooms, the same courses, the same student cafeterias, the same recreational activities over a period of days were enough to bring them together . . . These were the conditions for love at first sight, resulting in marriage!

Other encounters illustrate this apparently idyllic, unusual aspect which would seem to be due to nothing other than chance: 'It happened one evening at one of our choir practices. He was the friend of one of my friends in the choir' (Nurse, aged 27). Living and working in a rural area, not far from Brest, this nurse came to the weekly practices in search of friendship with the townspeople. She met a foreigner and started going out with him. They were married a few months later.

We met at a gathering at which the postgraduate students were having new lecturers introduced to them in the Arts Faculty at R. . ., in October 1966 . . . (French male lecturer, aged 38).

This lecturer married one of his students of the same age. She too then became a teacher in France where she had followed her husband. Having left when he was quite young to work in North West Africa, he was open to meeting to someone he would like.

We first met in the United States in the autumn of 1959, only two months after I arrived. My older sister knew my husband's family. We were students. He was eighteen, and I was seventeen (. . .) It wasn't until two years later that we really got to know one another when I was teaching him French and we started going out together in the summer of 1961 (French woman, aged 32, married to an American).

This French student, who is now an English teacher in a private establishment, married her white American husband. They live in central France where he works as a manager.

My older sister, who was married to an American, was instrumental in my own marriage and also in that of my other sister who is now married to an American (Idem).

Love at first sight may have been the determining factor in the encounter which ended in marriage for the older sister, but can we say the same for the marriages of the other two sisters?

Even if the encounter with the other person can, in some cases, have very unusual circumstances surrounding it, one has to recognise that there are sometimes other elements which greatly assist chance. Is not love at first sight itself often conditioned by unconscious mental images? These images are a reflection of the ego, and being so unusual and highly prized it suddenly erupts into desire.

These images may, depending on the nationality and type of person, be enhanced by favourable prejudices. The writer Virgil Georghiu, in one of his recent works, describes an encounter between a seminarist and a French woman[4]. In an interview with Jacques Paugam he gave the following reply:

A very beautiful woman, a beautiful woman, is a French woman, in common parlance . . . This truth is borne out in reality. Every day I am more convinced that true tenderness in this world is to be found in flowers, children, girls and the French woman (. . .) (Interview, *France-Culture*, 10th February 1978, broadcast on 'Prejudices').

Highly prized to the extreme, this 'French woman' is imbued with extraordinary qualities. Perhaps this is the image put across by some women in the upper classes where mixed marriages are unions which benefit from privileged conditions of existence. Comfort and a large income can be a great advantage to married life. However, many mixed marriages exist in less affluent circles.

With Algerians at least, it is mostly girls on social security, or from somewhat socially handicapped families, characterised by poverty or alcoholism. They were all breaking away from their families. Actually both partners are outcasts from their own groups and their union is a reflection of two rejections. The man has been rejected by Algeria. Now he's had to rent a single room; for that very reason he feels rejected by his community in France. And what do you expect a poor young girl to do with one room, alone, unemployed, unqualified . . . It is inevitable. The first encounter takes place and they both follow the same path; they live together in the same cramped accommodation. The same thing applies to students, on another level (Frenchman, aged 36, social worker).

The professional activities of this social worker bring him into constant contact with foreigners and mixed marriages. While acknowledging cohabitation before marriage as a factor which favours marriage, what he says reveals the existence of what are sometimes very clear social factors leading to the creation of mixed marriages. Although they are very often thought of as exceptions — with certain peculiar elements of their own — these marriages actually obey the same rules as marriages that are not mixed, as Alain Girard has described very well in his study on *Le Choix du Conjoint*[5] [The Choice of a Partner].

Nevertheless, an encounter between two foreigners sets in motion feelings of fascination and attraction which will be all the more intense and obsessive if the social pressure exerted by their respective groups is marked. The secret intimacy becomes a strong relationship in the face of a hostile environment. Moreover, it brings with it an element of risk and of the unknown. The partners in a mixed marriage are expressing their opposition to the social groups that wanted to 'pigeon-hole' them.

**Notes to Chapter 2**

1. Albin Michel, Paris 1964, 270 pp.
2. White American journalist who had his skin tinted in order to conduct a study on relationships between blacks and whites in the U.S.A.
3. A training scheme for young people out of work who, instead of just being registered as unemployed, take various courses with a view to making it easier for them to get into the job market.
4. *Le Grand Exterminateur* [The Great Exterminator], Plon, Paris, 1978.
5. Paris: PUF, 1974, 208 pp.

# 3 The reactions of the family

*'My daughter is in America!'*

'My daughter is in America'.
'My daughter is in Africa and wears a veil'.
'My brother has been converted to Islam'.
'They had a Jewish wedding'.

These remarks indicate enthusiasm and satisfaction on one side and, on the other side, regret, or bitterness, if not complete disagreement, compounded by the rift which can develop between a family and its loved one.

That's all the gratitude we got. After all we went through to bring her up we can't see her any more ... God knows when we will see her now! We haven't even met our grandson. We've seen a photograph of him, but how can you tell from a photograph whether he has more black blood in him or white (Frenchman whose daughter had married a black African).

In some countries and some social groups the wish of an individual to marry a foreigner takes on the dimensions of a scandal with all the consequences that that involves. Ingrid Bergmann, the world-famous actress, spoke in a literary programme on French television of all the indignation her second marriage to film producer Rossellini caused. The press in her country went as far as calling her a tart. The actress was quite clear: 'It was an Italian ... perhaps if he had been Swedish things would have been different'.[1] The fact that her new husband was Italian was a greater shock to Swedish public opinion than her divorce.

The journalist Henri Amouroux tells a harrowing tale in one of his books about something that happened in France during the occupation. The laws of the Vichy government forbade marriage with Jews. A certain doctor was against his son marrying a young Jewish student. Faced with the determination on his son's part, the doctor wrote to the German authorities, reporting his future daughter-in-law. She was arrested. Wanting at all costs to release his fiancée, and being unable to think of any other solution, the son told his father that the marriage was off. Together they went to the police to withdraw the complaint. They were told that she had already been sent to a concentration camp in Germany. Her parents were also arrested. The son was killed by the Germans because, following this painful affair, he had become involved in the Resistance movement.[2] This love story thus had a tragic end because the family, social and national environment cruelly stopped these two individuals from coming together. It was war and the Jews were the object of ruthless discrimination.

Claire Etcherelli, at the end of one of her fine books, tells of the disappearance of an Algerian who was in love with a French woman during the Paris repression at the time of the war with Algeria.[3] But more than ten years after the end of this war, it was learned that, because of the fierce opposition of her parents to her marriage with an Algerian intellectual, a French woman had committed suicide! Even if these specific examples are to be interpreted in a very unfavourable light, they are nevertheless indicative of the existence of certain real feelings of resistance.

The reactions to mixed marriages can be considered at a number of different levels. The reactions of the close family, those of friends and those of colleagues at work constitute circles of opposition of varying degrees of intensity. In addition to this, the district or town are also places in which mixed marriages will be tolerated to different degrees. Finally there is the overall opinion of the people of the country concerned and, more specifically, the opinions of social groups which will be made clear in their own particular ways for mixed couples of certain nationalities.

Marriage to a foreigner always upsets the existing equilibrium in a family, especially if this is the first of its kind in the immediate experience of the family. The parents and close family of the couple are the first to be involved and they have to take the often unfavourable comments of their relations and friends. These opinions will assume varying complexions depending on the religion, nationality and social status of the foreign partner. A white American son-in-law, working as an international official at UNESCO, will as a rule experience fewer difficulties in becoming accepted than another international official who comes from a Muslim country. Both of them, however, will experience less opposition than a skilled immigrant worker who, in addition to the difference in nationality (and possibly of religion) will also have a different social status. The accumulative effect of fairly hardened differences will directly

influence the opinions expressed within the family and among one's friends
and colleagues. How many fathers, when announcing that their daughter
is soon to marry a man from Senegal, have had to put up with comments
from long-standing friends such as: 'Oh, my dear chap, I'm sorry! The
monkey is always resurfacing in the Negro'. A classification of nationalities
and colours is always cropping up. The prospective foreign partner is
always prejudged in a good or bad light.

When confronted with a *fait accompli* some parents do all they can
to make the best of the situation: 'I said to my son-in-law: there's nothing
to worry about. You've married a French woman, so you are French. The
fact that you are black is of no importance as far as I am concerned'.

The desire at all costs to play down the difference that exists has its
origin in emotive feelings which develop from indifference to paternalism.
This sweeping aside of a reality quickly comes up against obstacles when
the man's son-in-law starts to look for a job in the town where all his
in-laws live. He was soon told that they feared there would be racist
reactions in a firm if he was employed at the level of his qualifications!
His son-in-law's diplomas would justify his looking for a middle management job. 'If only they'd taken him on to sweep the floors, no one would
have made a fuss!' So long as he poses no threat, a foreigner is accepted
or, at least, tolerated. In order not to create problems he must stay in the
place which the host group gives to him, both in terms of looking for a
job and when it comes to looking for a wife. This Senegalese had actually
crossed certain boundaries which the group was not used to seeing crossed.
'All the same, he's not just anyone. And if my daughter chose him . . . after
having turned down I don't know how many local lads!' Feeling useless
in Europe, she had gone to Africa on a VSO scheme. It was there that
she met her future husband.

All these reactions take their place in a graduated thinking system
which is not specifically that of her close family or friends alone, but that
of a far more universal context. These reactions are to be found in the very
nature of the relationship between a majority host population and foreign
minority populations.

In France the numerical size of foreign populations does not fully
explain a greater preference for one nationality over another. Nor does
it explain outright exclusion. The actual position a foreigner is allowed to
occupy depends to a large extent on his/her social position. Is he a doctor,
or an architect? If so, his social status will be favourably accepted. 'I
married a Moroccan architect'. In this case it is primarily the architect who
is being married and not the Moroccan. It would be quite a different

matter for a coloured man from Senegal who works as a cleaner on the railway in Paris. The social status of the individual will then be interpreted on the basis of rank in the hierarchy of sympathies according to nationality, colour, religion.

A study by INSED (the National Institute for Demographic Studies), carried out in 1971, clearly shows the different ways in which French people behave to foreigners depending on their origin. The Italians, the Spanish and the Portuguese were seen in a favourable light by the majority of people questioned; but the same people were more guarded in their views of people from N.W. Africa, black Africans, Turks and Yugoslavians. The dominant religion had more to do with this than nationality in establishing the distinction. Immigration from Latin countries (Italians, Spaniards, Portuguese) which are predominantly Christian was preferred to more recent immigration which was mostly Muslim. The geographical, cultural, religious and historical proximity of this earlier immigration did not alter the basic thought patterns.

Certain periods of history can have a decisive effect on whether marriages will occur. The two world wars for a long time prevented marriages between French and German people. Likewise the Algerian war practically precluded any union in a country where colonisation only favoured a few mixed marriages. Nevertheless sizeable communities lived alongside one another, some of them at close quarters in the towns with very similar standards of living. Although the census of 1906 in Algeria showed there to be significant numbers of different nationalities: approximately 450,000 of French stock, 117,000 Spaniards and 33,000 Italians,[4] there were very few mixed marriages. Only one in 1900, two in 1906, but 26 in 1907. It is only after 1930, Algeria's centenary, that any development of these figures occurred. According to the figures gathered by Dr Marchand, an estimated 75 marriages a year would seem to have been the maximum, for the whole of the Algerian territory, in the years between 1939 and 1953.

The same thing applied in France. When people first started to immigrate from Spain and Italy, a marked opposition was demonstrated. This disappeared with time. In this context, the example of the marriages between French and American people during the First World War is significant. Later on, the example of Franco-German marriages after the Second World War is also illuminating.

From 26th June 1917 to 20th October 1919, some 200,000 American soldiers were billeted in the Nantes/Saint-Nazaire region. Twenty thousand remained there permanently, against a local population of

220,000.[5] The presence of this military male population, in a very confined area, immediately resulted in marriages with the women of Saint-Nazaire and Nantes. Taking the town of Saint-Nazaire alone, with 130 Franco-American marriages, one in five marriages was mixed in 1919. The fact that many of the marriageable men from Saint-Nazaire had gone acted in favour of these marriages, as though they had left their places to the American soldiers who had occupied their territory. The reactions of the population were not always characterised by great feelings of sympathy towards the Allied soldiers. After the period of enthusiasm and infatuation which accompanied the hope engendered by the presence of these soldiers in a time of war, there followed a sense of disenchantment which was expressed openly to any French woman who had anything to do with the foreigners. Not only were they 'whores', they were also encouraging a dangerous growth in the practice of prostitution.[6] The people of Nantes, according to a police report, no longer wanted to see these 'gangs of girls and their pimps' on their streets. 'Are there no longer any honest women left in France?' asked the newspapers. Reactions were not all in this vein, of course. They did, after all, write a song to celebrate these mixed marriages between 'allies' [female] and 'allies' [male], certain verses of which demonstrate a mixture of humour and naive encounters:

We all know what to do to make ourselves understood.
Love doesn't know any national barriers
And its conversation is very tender (. . .)

And the eyes, taking the place of speech,
seemed to say, full of hope:
I love you — kiss me!
To be your husband
Dear little French woman (. . .)

At the last meeting they said:
— I take you as my wife, little French woman
— Dear ally, I take you as my husband.

All right! Beautiful!
Before the Mayor and the Consul
The valiant khakis will be
reunited with the daughters of France.
Long live the Alliance[7] (. . .)

Franco-German marriages were only possible some years after the Armistice: 423 in 1945 in France, they rose to 1347 in 1946 and 3937 in 1949[8]. The obstacles erected by the war between the two countries were real. All the reports concerning French women who had anything to do with the Germans leave little room for amorous passion. Again, one only has to read the writings of journalist Henry Amouroux.[9]

The recent reactions to marriage between French people and people from N.W. Africa are characteristic of this point of view on both sides of the Mediterranean. 'He's still only an Arab she picked up in the middle of Lent' (French businessman, in a provincial town).

This opposition from the French world to mixed marriages is nothing new, nor is it one-sided. It has its roots in colonialism and in the Algerian war; these only served to strengthen prejudices which were already firmly entrenched. They are exhibited equally in N.W. Africa itself, and often very violently. Here too the causes are complex. The women of the old colonial countries may feel they are being competed against when they see foreign women in the arms of their menfolk. This was the objection expressed in the statement of the UNFT (National Union of Tunisian Women) in December 1962:

> Is it right that students should enjoy themselves abroad with money from the national coffers which the whole of our people has earned by the sweat of its brow, and for them then to marry foreign women thereby robbing Tunisian women of the material wealth they deserve.[10]

Those women who have remained in their native land see themselves as downgraded by men returning from Europe with non-Muslim wives. When a student was in Europe, a mixed marriage could frustrate long-standing family plans. This was also the view taken by the President of Morocco, Allal-El-Fasi. More than twelve years later he confirmed this stance in an article entitled 'High officials and mixed marriage', which came out in 1974:

> Since Morocco gained its independence, a growing number of young Moroccan men are opting for mixed marriages, and in particular those who go to Europe to pursue their studies, thinking that the foreign woman is civilised, and will therefore be in a better position to help them solve the problems of life, and that the Moroccan woman has not yet reached the same level of emancipation and the required degree of maturity, making her incapable of meeting the requirements of modern man. Because of this, a group of eminent Moroccan personalities with foreign consorts has come into being, and these liaisons have given birth to 'halfcastes'. It is necessary that we call a spade a spade.[11]

This is a savage attack and it is couched in unambiguous terms. The
Moroccan leader is recalling certain aspects of Koranic doctrine in this
article. If the marriage of a Muslim man with a non-Muslim woman is
tolerated in many cases, the marriage of a Muslim woman with a
non-Muslim man is strictly forbidden, unless the latter is converted to
Islam. In all events any children born will become Muslim.

These purely religious obstacles are often supplemented by political
ones, The media frequently brings us reports on these 'marriages across
frontiers' which come up against all sorts of difficulties. Franco-Rumanian
couples can wait years before being granted the necessary marriage
permit. It was the personal intervention of French Prime Minister
Raymond Barre in talks with the Chinese Prime Minister Teng Hsiao Ping
which made possible the first Franco-Chinese marriage between Odile
Pierquin and Ti Han Li.

Even when all these obstacles are not raised, mixed marriages often
evoke a cautious response from public opinion. A survey carried out by
the journal *Croissance des Jeunes Nations*[12] [Growth of Young Nations]
produced some interesting findings. To the question: 'Are you in favour
of marriages between blacks and whites?', the responses varied from one
country to another:

| Response as a percentage | Yes | No | Don't know |
| --- | --- | --- | --- |
| Sweden | 67 | 21 | 12 |
| France | 62 | 25 | 13 |
| U.S.A. | 20 | 72 | 8 |

Countries such as Austria, Canada, West Germany, Norway,
Uruguay, Great Britain and the United States showed a majority opinion
against such marriages.

President Senghor — who himself married a French woman from
Normandy — advises that there should be a certain level of culture in
common for an interracial marriage to succeed. Philip Roth, in his book
*Portnoy et Son Complexe*[13] [Portnoy's Complaint], explains how mixed
Jewish marriages in America are a sign of acculturation and assimilation.

Opinions on mixed marriages can therefore be seen to vary from one
country to another. They may be very different depending on the period

in history through which a country has passed and on the time at which they are expressed. A clear-cut objection in one place may lose any real significance in another. For example, an Irish couple in which the husband is Catholic and the wife Protestant can live quite happily together in Paris, whereas they would be faced with all sorts of difficulties in Belfast where violent confrontations between the two communities often take place. In the same way it would be far easier for a mixed couple to live together in the built-up areas of some towns where the anonymity of relationships can be an advantage. This marriage would be the topic of every conversation in a small village in the heart of France where a stricter control is exerted. This same mental attitude to acceptance or rejection of the mixed couple is found in the U.S.A. between the states of the North and those of the South.

The acceptance of a mixed marriage between a French person and someone from N.W. Africa was seen as normal in France in a left-wing environment. That is until the day when the couple went through a crisis situation, accompanied by violence. Though they had been in favour when the couple first met, the friends quickly changed their minds about this type of marriage and found all sorts of reasons and arguments to justify and hasten the breaking off of the relationship.

The complex nature of such unions makes it impossible to identify a consistent set of opinions with respect to all mixed couples. We can only discern the general trend of reactions and attitudes in each particular context. The immediate family circle may have positive or negative reactions due to a social environment which to varying degrees does or does not accept such partnerships. Variations in the acceptance level may be observed depending on the religion, nationality, skin colour and social status of the foreign partner. A whole series of values, which will vary from one country to another, will predetermine the level of integration of the foreigner who has married a national, that is to say who has become a new member of the family and of the social group. American, Swiss, German, Iranian, N.W. African, West Indian or Senegalese, the partner will come before the new mother-in-law like a candidate at an examination. The difficulty of the test will depend on the foreigner's origin, and this will determine his or her ability to break into a group of people who share the same standards, values, complicities and interests. In cases of greatest conflict, the family will reject the foreign partner completely and will treat him or her with indifference. However, these initial attitudes may change with time.

A mother is first of all shocked to discover that her son is going out with a Jewish girl. But then she thinks to herself: 'She's pretty; and she's a musician. They met in the student choir. It's actually music which has brought them together'. She is reassured and, after the examination, the Jewish identity of her future daughter-in-law becomes secondary: 'After all, she's only Jewish on her father's side'. But she is anxious to find out from her son that they will have a proper wedding in a Catholic church, which they do.

As the days go by, fondness for this future daughter-in-law increases. The in-laws on both sides will meet, get to know one another, and express their opinions: 'They're very pleasant people; they gave us a marvellous reception'. Since they had never known any Jews and might even harbour traces of latent anti-semitism, the parents of the young man soon found themselves taking a summer holiday on a kibbutz in Israel: 'It's a very special sort of life, but you have to admit that these Jews have some remarkable qualities. When you think of all they went through during the war . . .' A splendid holiday at the initiative of their son and daughter-in-law who will often go to spend a summer holiday on a kibbutz.

The daughter-in-law is now fully integrated into the whole family, particularly among her sisters-in-law who see outstanding qualities in her. Everyone forgets that she is from a Jewish background. In the home of this young couple, however, there are clear signs of a living Jewish consciousness. Together, and in an intimate way, the two partners engage in a daily Judaeo-Christian search: this is a matter for the couple rather than for the families.

There had been nothing to prepare this traditional Catholic family for the assimilation of a Jewish girl. And yet certain positive elements — music, her physical appearance: 'She is pretty' — were helpful factors in allowing her to become completely integrated into the family circle. In a sense she has passed her entrance exam . . . But not all the tests are yet over! She is expecting a child. 'Will the baby be given a Christian baptism?' the parents wonder. They sincerely hope so.

The development of judgments is not always so easy. For instance, we see a retired couple who had always rejected their own daughter married to an African and living in Gabon for the last six years. She experienced many problems during the first few years of marriage. She and her partner separated twice and then came back together. A number of times she stayed in France with her children who were completely Negroid in appearance. After several years of hesitation she decided to live in Africa with her husband, even allowing a certain amount of polygamy on his part. One summer, with great apprehension, her parents went to visit her there. It came as a great surprise for them to discover that their daughter had adapted marvellously: 'She wasn't really made for living in France. Down there she can live life at her own pace and feels at home. Fortunately . . .' they now confide, as they confess their enthusiasm for this black Africa about which they only knew the classic stereotypes before their trip, ideas passed on from colonial days. They have changed because of the unexpected positive development they have seen in their daughter: 'When she was in France, she always had problems and could never settle down to anything'.

Each couple can develop its own strategy for gaining recognition in each partner's group of origin. One couple, for instance, presented their situation first to an influential older sister who would gradually, over a period of months, announce the planned marriage of her sister to a foreigner, taking each member of her hostile family one by one. She spoke to them all, countering the barrage of arguments they raised, and took advantage of the inevitable interrelationships and the dynamics of the family. An event like this could not have been accepted all at once. Time for 'converting' the environment was needed.

But some situations remain unresolved.

You just have to get used to the French family. You have to find the right words, the right language if you want to communicate, and it's not easy. As for my own family, their reactions were very negative. They wouldn't speak to me about it. I left Algeria angry (Algerian woman married to a French man).

Some reactions can be so antagonistic that they involve extreme attitudes. This was the case, for example, when a young Muslim girl was simply sent back to her country of origin. This young Algerian girl was going out with a French boy. When he found out about it, her father put her on a plane back to Algeria that very week. Many such disputes are being dealt with by juvenile courts. Mainly they affect the young daughters of immigrant workers who have been settled in France for some years. These girls find it difficult to find their own identity between their personal needs and the requirements of their parents. These difficult cases often add to crises of adolescence and differences of opinion over matters of the heart.

There was a brief moment of surprise (sudden marriage), and perhaps also for my father a reaction against the fact that we were a mixed couple. For him it is very important to maintain and even to support the basic values of our French society, values which he has seen being

eroded over the years (music, dress). My father is — how can I put
it — a sort of nationalist communist. There may therefore have been
a moment of surprise for him. But everything's sorted out now,
although there have been problems (Frenchman, student of architecture, married to a Muslim woman).

This student, from a working class family, expresses how his marriage
was received. Every summer on an Atlantic beach he would meet this
young girl from a devout N.W. African business family.

My family's reaction was very accommodating from the moment my
husband showed a willingness to become a Muslim. It is obligatory
by law in our country that both marriage partners be Muslim,
especially in the case of the husband. Apart from that it is not
particularly difficult. It was enough for him to affirm this by repeating
a phrase. This gesture made it possible for us not to shock anyone and
to keep good family relations, as well as enabling us to resolve all the
problems which can arise when a woman marries a non-Muslim
(Muslim woman, married to the French student above).

This woman is referring to the formula known as the shahada — the
profession of faith in Islam — which is recited in order to declare oneself
a Muslim. This formality was necessary here in order for the foreign
partner to be admitted to the religious group of his wife, although it is not
required for a woman (Christian or Jewish) who marries a Muslim man.

All the examples of couples we have referred to above show multiple
variations of experience depending on the cultures, religions, countries
and points in time involved. The foreign partner thus goes through a sort
of entrance examination which may be quite legalistic and formal where
it has to do with official institutions. This is not always the case with the
close family and social group which tends to exercise a continuous control.
This integration of the foreign partner is never total or final. He must pass
a number of tests in order to gain full recognition from his wife's family,
as is the case with all husbands. But in the case of mixed marriages the
nature of the tests will involve the very nature of the bond and
commitment to the group. This social control is exercised over the
foreigner on a continual basis, as well as over both partners in general and,
later, over their children who will become the crucial social bond: children
will bring the couple into even stricter conformity with the group if they
had in any way moved away from it. It is often the mother-in-law who
takes the part of examiner and who then, implicitly or explicitly, decides
whether the foreign partner is to be admitted to the group which she then
undertakes to convince of her decision. The whole family takes it upon

itself to announce this new admission and to inform their immediate social group. From being a candidate, the partner now becomes a graduate whose qualities are praised. He is made a member of a group which will recognise his abilities, qualities and rights. The marriage has now become an event and not just an 'intimate affair' between two individuals. At the same time it has an effect, in successive waves, on the whole of the social fabric, and changes it. Acting as an indicator of the true structures of the group, this marriage will put the bonds between the group members to a searching test. By creating new bases, it will cause fragile or superficial bonds to crack open, whilst creating new bonds of solidarity and reinforcing already existing relationships which will be renewed as a result of it. Whereas it could be something which weakens the members or even destroys the whole group, it can also become a factor which encourages greater cohesion. In the context of the overall social scene this marriage has a high profile for every one who comes into contact with it. It will always act as a reminder of a test which the group has had to go through and from which it may have suffered. The social identity has been at stake. What will it mean for the future of the group — something to be proud of, or something which causes the group to be excluded, disqualified and isolated by other groups?

## Notes to Chapter 3

1. Antenne 2, *Apostrophes*, 26th September 1980.
2. *La Vie des Français Sous l'Occupation* [The Life of the French during the Occupation]. Paris: Fayard, 1961, p.399.
3. *Élise ou la Vraie Vie* [Elise, or the True Life]. Paris: Denoël, 1967, 284 pp.
4. Source: Algerian Statistical Yearbook, new series.
5. Source: Yves-Henri Houailhat, *Les Americains à Nantes et à Saint-Nazaire* [The Americans in Nantes and Saint-Nazaire]. Literary Annals of the University of Nantes, Fine Arts, Paris, 1977.
6. *Le Travailleur de l'Ouest* [The Worker of the West], 27th April 1918.
7. Dupre de la Roussiere, *Nantes Mondain*, November 1917.
8. Source: INSEE, civil records.
9. One might also look at *La Tondue* [The Shorn One] by G. Groussy. Paris: Le Seuil, 1980.
10. *La Presse*, 9th January 1963, Tunis.
11. *El Alam*, French edition: *L'Opinion* [The Opinion]. Rabat 13th May 1916 and 17th March 1974.
12. No. 118, December 1971, pp. 34–35.
13. Gallimard, Paris 1970, 280 pp.

# 4 A constant historic fact

*'Still in Ancient Greece!'*

The construction of Europe seems to be an important political preoccupation and the election of a Parliament based on universal suffrage has created an official political institution. But bonds have already been woven between the men and women of all these different countries. Europeans marry other Europeans, and what is more they marry non-Europeans, mainly migrants and foreign students. For decades now mixed couples have been experiencing the difficult day-by-day reality one can well imagine when one thinks of the diversity and even the contradictions of the laws governing nationality.

What is true today for such marriages has also been the case throughout history for other groups of countries. In 1979 the Nine countries of the EEC contained a significant Catholic block with Belgium, France, Italy and Luxembourg. Spain and Portugal were later to strengthen this European Catholic element. Great Britain (90% Anglican), Denmark (97% Lutheran) and West Germany (51% Protestant) also form another religious block. We should not forget Ireland, 75% Catholic, where a great many religious and economic rifts coincide. Marriages between people of different denominations have posed serious problems for the churches which are always trying not to lose their own members. In Europe of the future mixed marriages, as well as religious and national combinations, will not come about with any degree of lasting certainty, at least in the first instance, without hitting a number of cultural, legal and linguistic barriers. The Flemish–Walloon dispute is always resurfacing as an indication of a real sense of unease.

Nevertheless the figures for the last three decades reveal one truth: they may appear insignificant, but taken together they are striking. The 1968 census carried out by INSEE[1] identified 237,000 homes in which one of the partners was Italian by birth, 132,000 in which one of the partners was Spanish by birth and 78,000 marriages in which one of the partners was a Pole. The table below enables us to see the present extent of this phenomenon: there were more than 20,000 mixed marriages in France in 1981 alone.

By marriage and eventually naturalisation, the foreigner is integrated into a country which is not his own. He adds a sort of 'emotional and civil qualification' to a professional qualification when he has a job. Many foreign immigrants follow this pathway to integration. The children born to these couples settle on the basis of the country in which their parents take up residence. This was the case for thousands of couples. In the second generation, the children became French.

MIXED MARRIAGES IN FRANCE (FOR 1981)

| Nationality of the foreign partner | French husband | French wife | Totals |
|---|---|---|---|
| Algerian | 1,002 | 1,556 | 2,558 |
| German | 484 | 345 | 829 |
| Belgian | 272 | 411 | 683 |
| Spanish | 1,429 | 1,289 | 2,718 |
| Italian | 718 | 1,666 | 2,384 |
| Polish | 349 | 97 | 446 |
| Portuguese | 1,619 | 1,705 | 3,324 |
| Yugoslavian | 101 | 176 | 277 |
| Other nationalities | 2,283 | 4,816 | 7,099 |
| Totals | 8,257 | 12,061 | 20,318 |
| Percentages | 40.6 | 59.4 | 100 |

(Source: INSEE civil records table)

A number of official and private bodies seem to be recognising this newly emerging 'Europeanness'. There are bilateral associations that are organising exchanges, trips and residential language courses, such as the OFAJ (the Franco-German Youth Association). Movements between very close countries are increasing: at the same time they widen the boundaries of the 'endogamous circle' which, as L. Henry defines it, is the group of young unmarried who are likely to marry. The chances for foreigners to meet one another are now far greater. Alongside this we have the stratification of the European job market, on the one hand, and the increase in student and holiday migrations on the other. Even though the search for employment is the main objective, it also takes place at a time when the people concerned are young and therefore marriageable. Whether consciously or not, it is accompanied by the search for a partner. Contact between foreigners is furthermore facilitated by the rapid development of means of transport, railway links with neighbouring countries and air links with more distant countries.

The typical course taken by people who immigrate for financial reasons begins with the search for employment. It is in this way that they gain professional integration. If this stage is successful, they will perhaps consider settling down in the new country. From one stage of integration to another they may achieve emotional integration by marrying a member of the majority group. But these marriages do not always bring together people who are completely alien to one another. In such mixed marriages, for instance, one often discovers a difference of nationality, but not of religion. This is the case with Catholic immigrants from Mediterranean countries who have come and married a French national. The difference of the social environment is not always important. Foreign workers in France have a greater chance, statistically, of meeting young working class French people. The UNESCO official, on the other hand, will come into contact with a more well-to-do type of person. Very clear types of mixed marriage can therefore be seen to develop: between students, marriages in the working classes, marriages in the professions, marriages between international officials, between business people, in the medical/social world, etc. The same rules for the formation of a marriage can therefore be seen to apply as those for unions between people of the same nationality: the rules across national frontiers. According to the research carried out by A. Girard and L. Roussel, only one marriage in two in France took place between people from the same social group.

It will require great creativity at all levels to enable European (and other) couples to come up with mixed ways of conducting their daily lives. The attempts at political unity need to be supplemented by research which will harmonise the civil and religious jurisdictions, not to mention the education programmes. There will also be the need for a general willingness to get rid of the old stereotypes which still plague foreign partners in mixed marriages. A bad television film on the 1939–45 war exasperated a Franco-German couple when the word 'Boche' was used in every other sentence, perpetuating an unbearable antagonism by means of a cliché . . . 'It's always the same . . . As though there were not a large number of Germans who also died in concentration camps!' the German husband complains angrily to his French wife. They then have to switch off the set when their children join in by saying: 'That means we're "half-Boche"!' The confusion between Nazi and German still produces reactions which we are still far from erasing from our collective conscious. This persistent hatred for the 'Boche' has very old roots and is sadly responsible for behaviour characterised by rejection: 'As far as my family was concerned my grandmother, for instance, whose husband died as a result of the 1914–18 war, didn't want to come to my wedding (. . .). Afterwards, when she got to know my wife, she found her charming and delightful. But it took some time (. . .).' This French listener, married to a German woman, explained during a radio broadcast how he had lived in Berlin with his wife and children. His wife is now completely accepted by his parents, but at the time of his wedding, the German woman still represented the hereditary enemy.[2]

These few examples of European marriages nevertheless act as indicators of the actual conditions under which European marriages exist. Furthermore they may be seen ·as a challenge to national identity when it is perceived as a static reality. Thus, in addition to the political and economic alliances, these marriages are for the most part a concrete expression of relations between the different countries of Europe today.

But what about yesterday? In the distant past mixed marriages were also a serious issue, sometimes encouraged, but more often forbidden, or strictly regulated, especially in periods of conflict.

The Jewish people, during their exile, would not tolerate these marriages which weakened their identity in a threatening environment where they were in the minority. All minority communities, at one time or another, formulate laws to restrict the marriage of their members to outsiders. Is this not still the concern of certain intellectual Jews, particularly in the U.S.A.? They are not in favour of 'this lack of substance' which results from marriage to a non-Jew.[3] On the subject of American Jews, the concept of safeguarding a special identity is in opposition to the concept of complete assimilation. This is brought out in Roger Ikor's novel, *Les Eaux Melées*[4] [The Mixed Waters]. This book tells the story of a family of Jewish immigrants from Russia, which is completely assimilated into the French population. They forget their roots and make every effort to conform. The son, Simon, rejects his parents and his Jewish name. He marries in church. The daughter, Clara, marries a foreigner and her nephew becomes a Protestant minister after his conversion to Christianity. The father is happy to see his children completely assimilated into Christian society. The author completely opposes the romantics of the American Jewish school, such as Philip Roth, who, despite criticising

Jewish society, remain firmly in support of it. The Americans blame the French Jews for allowing themselves to be enticed away by the great assimilating force of French culture.

We see the same thing in Algeria today where the very strong Berber minority of Kabylia exercises a certain degree of endogamy so as to ensure thereby that their language will be passed on:

> For us Kabyles it would be out of the question for our women to marry outside of the group. A woman who marries a foreigner is a woman lost to the community, and to our language. And since we are a threatened community, we are not in favour of mixed marriage, even with Arab speakers (Man, aged 35 years, teacher).

Nevertheless, many Kabyle men marry outside of the group, urged on by an emigration which has lasted a number of decades, as they are forced out of a very poor region.

In Ancient Greece mixed marriages were a subject for debate. In the time of Pericles, in the year 450 BC, it was necessary to have an Athenian father in order to become a citizen. Thus it was possible to encounter aristocratic Athenians born of a foreign mother, e.g. Clisthenes or Themistocles. The law of Pericles in 451–450 BC removed this privilege and stipulated that henceforth only the children of an Athenian father and an Athenian mother would be classed as citizens. Even if this law was often stretched to the limit, it was nevertheless often referred back to. Only a few privileged individuals with but one Athenian parent were able to become citizens themselves. This was rarely the case for foreign groups, even among those who had fought for Athens. The population of the city was sharply divided between citizens, 'foreigners', and slaves. These social barriers were protected by a legislative system which did not tolerate marriage between the groups. The citizens were Athenians. The 'foreigners' were free men, Greeks and non-Greeks; being foreign in origin they had to pay a tax which 'indicated their inferior status to that of the citizens'.[5] The slaves had no rights. This organisation of legal and social barriers between groups within the population preserved the ethnic homogeneity on which the democracy of Ancient Greece was built. Since marriage with foreigners was forbidden, this also guaranteed the protection of landed property: only the Athenian citizens had the right to possess land.

At the time of the occupation of Calais (in the sixteenth century), the English mixed with the peoples of the north of France. Previously, during the wars between the two countries, the English kings did not allow their soldiers to marry French women except in rare cases. Under the Old Government, although there was a high birth rate, the population of France was slow in growing. The kingdom only succeeded in maintaining an adequate number of subjects by periodically welcoming foreigners who became part of the country's population. Many diplomats, artists, travellers, colonists, ship's captains, etc., married in the countries they visited and 'then returned to France bringing with them English, Italian, German, Indian or black women as wives; by means of the introduction of these foreigners, they contributed towards mixing the French population'.[6]

Even today there is legislation in some countries restricting such marriages. A high price was exacted from a couple who were found dead in their apartment in South Africa on 24th August 1978: they were Miss Bubbles M'Pondo, a well-known black model and her white fiancé of only a few months, Mr Jannie Beetge. They made a public announcement of their intention to marry, despite the apartheid laws which forbade this and proscribed any sexual relations between individuals of different races. Before their deaths, one bullet each in the head, they had been given an eight month suspended prison sentence.[7]

There were a number of press articles on the Soviet chess player, Spassky, in 1975. It was not until 1978 that he was granted French nationality, although he had left his own country two years earlier to live in Paris with his wife, a French woman he had met when she was a secretary at the French commercial bureau in Moscow. As in other cases, this marriage had its political repercussions.

With a certain amount of exaggeration, no doubt, the Chinese News Agency announced on 30th November 1976 that there were twenty thousand Soviet spies in France: 'The U.S.S.R., continued the Chinese News Agency, is receiving information through women of Soviet origin who have acquired the nationalities of various western countries. By way of example, an Italian weekly estimates that two thousand Soviet women have become Italian citizens through marriage. Many of them (. . .), provide the Soviet Union with information'.[8] The Press also devoted sensational coverage to the marriage of Christina Onassis to a Soviet official, Mr Kausov. They made a conspiracy, a real-life spy story, out of the affair. They tried to make of this marriage the seizure by the Kremlin of part of the Greek merchant fleet inherited by the young woman from her millionaire ship-owning uncle. Mr Kausov was portrayed as nothing more than a KGB seducer, and the adventuress, Christina, was seen as having fallen into the trap. The spectacular romance came to an end some months after the airing of these fanciful theories.

Whenever two foreigners are brought together in marriage, various things are at stake: these can be economic, political, religious or to do with the individual families. At the national level, this creates difficulties for all states. Even in France, Article 13 of the 1945 Decree stipulated that the marriage of a foreigner who was a temporary resident could only be celebrated if a government permit was first obtained. These legal provisions were not repealed until 1982.

But the legal aspects are not the only ones. These only serve to reflect a majority population's relations with individuals or foreign groups within its territory. They clearly show us the status of the foreigner over the course of history. In the sixteenth and seventeenth centuries, when Europe was divided up into Catholic and Protestant, there were strict laws prohibiting the marriage of people of different confessions. These lasted a very long time and posed serious problems for the families of the couple to be, as well as for the political authorities when there was much at stake on these marriages. The marriage of Count Henri Laborde de Monpezat to Princess Margrethe of Denmark in 1966 is significant in this respect. A number of articles appeared in the national and international Press. This was the marriage of a Catholic to a Protestant. But the social status of the Protestant princess meant that she was destined to succeed to the highest position in Denmark, namely that she would in a few years become queen of that country. As soon as the engagement was confirmed, they announced the decision of the Count de Monpezat to become a Protestant. The Vatican gave its consent for him to settle his personal religious situation. Even Francois Mauriac gave his point of view in his leader article in the *Figaro Littéraire*. There was a short engagement, followed by the announcement of the wedding date and the plans for conversion. The wedding took place with royal pomp. A few years later they came to France on an official visit (December 1975). Not only was Count Henri now a fully-fledged Protestant, he was also referred to as Prince Henrik. He accompanied Queen Margrethe II, with their children who were also Protestants. Thus the succession to the throne was assured with religious legitimacy fully in keeping with the traditions of Denmark which will only accept Protestant sovereigns. Great Britain has also added fuel to debates on this subject when the marriage plans of the descendants of the Royal Family are discussed.

These examples of marriages could leave one thinking that only people who exercise political or symbolic responsibilities experience difficulties in becoming part of an established society. But many foreign partners do find their place in a national population through naturalisation. After having become more or less accepted in the family group, the foreign partner has to undergo various tests in order to achieve a national qualification. Often, when his or her place of residence has become more or less fixed, he or she will be ready to 'cross over', in order to become part of the group. This stage, which is very much like admission formalities, is an important indication of membership of a 'club'.

There may be many instances of naturalisation and they may be seen as a desirable thing. But do they in any way justify the ideology of cross-breeding? As far as genetics is concerned, as we saw earlier, diversity is a desirable characteristic, according to the experts. But naturalisations (as with mixed marriages) may seem to point to a cultural cross-breeding which is aimed at ironing out any religious, ethnic or linguistic difference, and this precisely at a time when a striking regionalism is appearing, both in Europe where, in France alone, there are the peoples of Brittany, Corsica, the Occitanian region, and the Walloon region, etc., and in N.W. Africa the Berbers and the Kabyles, not to mention other places in the world, e.g. the Druze and the Kurds, etc. Under these conditions mixed marriages pose new problems for the societies of today. Once societies have drawn up their own rules aimed at the reproduction of the groups from which they are formed, mixed marriages will be seen as a challenge to those rules for the orderly functioning of societies in that they bring together individuals who remain at the edge of their original groups. They will incur general disapproval in proportion to the extent to which they alter the nature of existing groups whose aims are to perpetuate themselves.

With the social identity and the reproduction of the groups themselves put at risk, it is not surprising that strict rules have been enforced to limit such cross-breeding. One must not forget that to marry a foreigner, that is to say someone who is different, means to violate the sexual taboo which is one of the most powerful factors in the normal identity of each group.

This is one of the arguments sometimes launched, in the form of extremist slogans, by ruthless supporters of nationalist ostracism: 'Soon they will be sleeping with your women!' When a person who is different tries to gain admission to a group, they arouse distrust and suspicion. They pose a threat to a social group and the latter responds with undisguised aggression. This is because the group does not want to become too readily accessible, for fear of being too vulnerable. It will draw up all possible defences, all the psychological barriers available to it in order that its integrity, on which its identity is based, may not be breached. This arsenal of defence mechanisms may take on xenophobic connotations, it may even be completely racist in nature, in response to immigration from N.W.

Africa, for example, in which Mr Le Pen, the President of the National Front in France, sees 'the advanced guard of the Barbarians launching their attack on the West'.[9]

As soon as it is no longer exceptional, mixed marriage becomes a social phenomenon and, soon, a problem. But is it so different from marriages which are not 'mixed'? Does it not take place with the same intentions in mind? It would seem to be a marriage in which one can only justifiably speak of its mixed nature in terms of special distances introduced by religion and culture. Is not every marriage a mixed one? Is it not only the nature and intensity of the differences between the two partners which determine how great the mix is? Given these circumstances, does the mixed couple confirm the importance of the institution of marriage, or does it, on the contrary, reveal it to be secondary to love? 'Must it not be the case that people who to begin with were foreigners to one another need to have a great deal of love in order to get married?' One thus attempts to justify mixed marriage by stressing the unusual intensity of love required. But people in mixed marriages also get divorced, as do people in other marriages. It would seem then that to speak of feelings, in this case, serves only to mask the social reality.

Can people, who are foreigners to each other in terms of religion, race, nationality, colour and language, etc., really contemplate a shared life while remaining foreigners? Would they not be forced to recognise the 'foreignness' of their partner? Starting out from this dynamic recognition of the differences and identities of each partner, they will need to come up with a way of living together which both of them can accept.

Moreover, is not the mixed couple an extreme version of all couples in which one can clearly see the whole range of interactions between people in relationships of this type? We can look on it as a test case, a sort of laboratory or stage for marital relationships where it is impossible to escape basic questions in such extreme conditions. It is actually the privileged and difficult setting for an encounter between two people faced with the task of living out a lasting intensity of feelings in an environment which is not prepared to allow them to enjoy this experience ... To varying degrees mixed marriages clearly show us factors which may lie hidden in marriages which are not mixed.

**Notes to Chapter 4**

1. Institut National des Statistiques et des Études Economiques.

2. *France-Inter*, a broadcast by Ève Ruggieri on mixed marriages, 6th November 1980.
3. A book on this subject by G. Friedmann, *Fin du Peuple Juif* [End of the Jewish People]. Paris: Gallimard, 1965. 376 pp.
4. Albin Michel, Paris 1956, 314 pp.
5. Michel Austin and Pierre Vidal-Naquet, *Économies et Sociétés en Grèce Antique* [Economies and Societies in Ancient Greece]. Paris: Colin (U2), 1972, p. 116.
6. J. Mathorez, *Foreigners in France under the Old Government* (Vol. I). Paris: Old Lib. Édouard Champion, 1919, p. 129.
7. *Le Monde*, 26th August 1978.
8. *Le Monde*, 2nd December 1976.
9. *Le Monde-Dimanche*, 19/20th September 1983.

# Part 2
# The Relationship of a Couple

# 5 The male and female roles

*'We are quite different'*

*'It is true, we are different, you are a woman and I am a man'*.
The great difference right at the start is precisely this. It is what distinguishes a man and a woman in the same group, not only physically, but also socially and culturally. It will always be present in the journey which the two partners undertake together. It is not only a fundamental distinction, it will also be coloured, accentuated and defined by each partner's culture, religion and social environment.

It is impossible to equate a white woman who is a university professor in Pittsburgh and married to a black man who is also a university professor, with a white woman married to a black worker living in an apartment in a working class area. The Jewish woman married to a Catholic living in New York, in a structured community which is reviving Jewish traditions, cannot be compared with a young Jewish woman who is married to a Catholic but living in Rennes, Brittany.

The images of men and women have been sharply defined by societies which have divided up tasks, work and even space. Is one not struck, for instance, when walking around in Arab towns of the Middle East at the end of the afternoon, to see in the streets large crowds consisting solely of men, the women being at home preparing the evening meal? Is there not also a division of time and space? On the doors of Turkish baths one sees signs which read 'time reserved for women'.

This intimate experience of sexual differences will be transferred and exist alongside the cultural differences between a mixed couple. Being an unusual couple among other 'ordinary' couples they will, by their internal dynamics, reveal what goes on, to a less intense degree, in all couples where there are differences, be they obvious or subtle. Indeed the mixed couple can act as a mirror of what is to be found in all couples.

At the start of their life together, above all, the partners of a mixed marriage will be likely to experience, with greater intensity, the novelty of an encounter between two people of different nationalities. Moreover this novelty is supplemented by an element of the original and unusual. They are aware that they are not only 'alone in the world' but that they are 'alone in the world in a different way' in comparison with all the other couples they come into contact with. They realise that they are in some way exceptions in an environment which maintains its expected rules of conduct, and with which these other couples have complied. As we have already seen, the reactions of people around them will not all be positive. On the contrary, there will often be fierce opposition. The effect of all these factors will be to strengthen the bond which unites them. They therefore have a tendency to isolate themselves from all social contexts and to live in a neo-romantic style, placing a high value — sometimes too high a value — on what unites them, and playing down what, objectively, separates them. They live a life centred on themselves, perhaps reaching the point of wanting to prove and justify the validity of this 'love relationship'. This will be even more the case if the partners had previously had unhappy experiences with other partners.

Sometimes exhibiting the psychological behaviour of outcasts, cut off from their respective environments, they will put much into their relationship and feelings. Being excluded from society will only serve to bring them closer together. They will exist in a limited circle of friends rather than in their families who, being more closely affected by the couple's intentions, will have less disinterested reactions than their friends will! The partners will tend to place too great a value on this relationship of love if they are opposed on two fronts. Indeed they often unite against their respective groups but, in addition, these groups are opposed to one another. Their marriage becomes a real challenge and it then seems the right thing to do to encourage this romantic union. In the light of the disapproving reactions of society, it becomes for them a highly valued private act. They are caught up in impossible realms of love, modelled on Romeo and Juliet, separated by social, national, religious and racial barriers. The partners will make every effort to overthrow these barriers. Sensational articles in the Press address this fascination with romantic love, with cases such as the marriage between a prince and a shepherd-girl (it is rarely a shepherd and a princess). This was the case with Aurélie, a French woman from a poor home who married the nomad prince of the Tidjania tribe in southern Algeria.

Many marriages do not reach this level of fame, however. Their neo-romanticism is a mask — perhaps a necessary one to begin with. It conceals a reality, but will perhaps make it possible to prolong the encounter stage of the relationship. Behind this veil, real differences exist between the partners and between the groups from which they come.

The distances are both objective and, sometimes, merely subjective ones. They may be conscious or quite unconscious differences. Whether the relationship is new or well established, these distances may be obvious, revealed, or more subtly hidden and lying dormant. They will be more or less noticeable, depending on when and where they are displayed, and they may be bearable at one moment and unbearable at another, then becoming the cause of conflicts which may serve the purpose of clearing the air and reducing them or, in contrast, of adding more fuel and driving a wedge between the partners.

Marriages between the French and people from N.W. Africa, a frequent occurrence in France, is a good example of marriages which present a series of fundamental distances and areas of opposition. These clearly reveal the areas in which there is a sharp contrast between the people coming together, at least at the cultural and religious levels. Experienced at the level of the partners themselves, these differences have their roots in the whole range of distances which actually exist between France and N.W. Africa. What constitutes a distance between individuals is the concentrated reflection of a real social distance between their respective social groups. The geographic distances alone place France in the moderate European continent, while N.W. Africa is used to various changes in climatic conditions, but it is frequently hotter than France. A partner who was born and spent the first twenty years of his life in a town in the South of Algeria where the torrid heat of the sun was a part of everyday life, may experience difficulties, in their physical being, when they try to adapt to the North of France. There will be a psychological cost to pay for changing their original metabolism. Endless grey, rainy days could cause them to withdraw into a world of nostalgia and into feeling an exile from their native country. Alongside this geographic transplantation, they may also be affected by olfactory and culinary changes. To eat a foreign dish for the first time may be enjoyable as a new experience, but when one's body is repeatedly subjected to foreign food, without the occasional reminder of one's traditional fare, this can have a conscious or unconscious adverse effect on the individual concerned and may lead to a slight feeling of lost identity. This is experienced by all exiles. In *A Day in the Life of Ivan Denisovitch*, Solzhenitsyn clearly evokes this sense of longing for the taste of soup from his native country. One may try one's own hand at cooking, but there will be limits. One's body is inescapably tied to a rhythm of work; the foreign man may now work in a metal works, whereas originally he could have been a nomadic shepherd at the edge of the Sahara. To move from a rural rhythm to an urban one can result in breakdowns at the physical level. In the early part of this century, research into 'the techniques of the body' by the ethnologist Marcel Mauss identified a number of cultural and social phenomena relating to the body as an overall social instrument and modelled by the individual's society of origin. When forced to adapt to different time and space parameters, the body will have to 'pay the price' and the repercussions may appear in the form of fatigue, ill humour, sexual drive, etc., which one partner may exhibit towards the other. The body is like an envelope, a concentration of the whole social and cultural heritage of rhythms, rites, taboos . . . and desires. I was told one day by a Muslim that he 'missed the Turkish baths' of his childhood. He then described all the pleasure he had experienced, when he was still young, of going with his mother and watching all the women and girls busily discussing every subject under the sun in that heat which causes extreme perspiration. Later on, in adult life, he became a devotee of the practice of taking Turkish baths; he found the western bathroom a poor and uninteresting substitute: 'places where you could get clean and yet remain impure'. He then went on to explain the religious connotations of the Turkish bath: a place of purification and ritual. As a committed Muslim he felt as though part of him had been amputated because it was impossible here to meet needs which were regarded as quite natural in his own country.

The couple will also be affected by the distances caused by the economic differences between France and N.W. Africa. These separate an industrialised country with a high level of average consumption from a country which is still developing, for the most part rural, and where consumption is low.

This aspect may be come across in minor details, such as throwing things away, nicely concealed in dustbins. 'To throw away bread' may seem an insignificant thing to do in France, though much more so in towns than in the country. However, it is contrary to all practice in N.W. Africa where parents teach children that a piece of bread, even if it is very dry, must never be left lying about, and certainly not just thrown away. We see combined here the economic factor and the symbolic, not to say sacred, investment related to a type of food.

'I just cannot understand how my wife can throw bread away; I find it disgraceful' (Muslim, aged 33).

But these economic distances will have other effects; one of the partners realises that he or she is a member of that group of people which, through lack of work or the lack of facilities for study in their own countries, have decided to emigrate. They also know that although foreign workers have a privileged status in their own country, they themselves have a precarious status which may end in unemployment, and even in 'pressure to return home'. There are also political distances: notions of liberty will be looked at differently when they are directly bound up with historical differences and the experience of colonialism. History has left its mark and the intimate relationship of a married couple may at times be affected, to an extent, especially when marital conflicts arise, by the old unequal relationship between the dominant race and the subjected people. This being the case, the partner from a country which used to be in subjection and is now seeking a new identity, will be readily attracted by various aspects of the former colonial power. This search, and we can see it in N.W. Africa, is a return to an intense Arabisation. Although bilingual in most cases, the partner will be aware of a complex social reality in Arabic or Berber, with nuances which his French partner will not be able to grasp. Unless a high cost is paid in terms of effort and time, whole areas of Muslim and Berber culture will remain unknown to the other partner. If that partner wants to learn Arabic, assuming the couple live in France, he or she will encounter far greater obstacles than the N.W. African partner would in perfecting his or her French, a language which will already be familiar from primary school and which will have been mastered to a great extent. All this will serve to introduce misunderstandings into the relationship which the French partner will not be able to accept because he or she will not always understand them.

The religious difference is one of the most important, even if the partners have decided to forget their religions. Because of pressure from in-laws, there will be periodic returns to certain practices. Some barriers are never completely crossed. The Muslim partner on holiday in N.W. Africa during the fast of Ramadan will find it difficult to fight the urge to do what everyone else is doing, i.e. to identify with their original community. The search for Islamic–Christian dialogue remains an initiative reserved for a privileged few who have the means and time to consider such matters. These cannot help but be enriched and encouraged by Islamic–Christian talks over the last few years in Tripoli and, above all, in Cordoba.

Nevertheless fierce opposition exists on both sides. Let us not forget, by way of example, the restrictions placed on Franco-Muslim marriages, as illustrated in the Dalila Maschino affair. This young woman, married to a non-Muslim Frenchman was 'returned to her family' in the spring of 1978 by her brother, aided by their sisters, when she was in Quebec. After having been married to a Muslim Algerian and made to stay with his family for three years in the village of El-Eulma (Algeria), she rejoined her first husband in Canada in the spring of 1981. Alongside the colonial distrust of Islam one needs to place longstanding distrust taught by the Christian churches. The search for dialogue between the religions is very recent and has not yet profoundly changed the way people think.

There are also differences in terms of what constitutes a family when one partner has been brought up in a large family and the other in a nuclear family where there is greater interchange of partners' roles. One child will have learned to depend on the sole authority of the parents and the family will have been the setting for a triangular expression of love and feelings. Whereas for the partner who was brought up in a different emotional world with a large number of uncles, aunts and cousins, under the watchful eyes of grandparents, this person will be familiar with looking on the home as a privileged place for social interaction.

Finally, a couple will be affected by differences in status and role (male and female) whose presence will be felt. A certain amount of progress, linked with the economic context and with feminism, has changed the place and role of women in Europe. Outside professional activity is making possible an ever increasing independence. It is causing people to think again about domestic chores, cooking and the number of children one will have and how they will be educated. The social nature of the intimate relationship of a couple is changing. The status of the mother is now less dominant, whereas it remains as strong in the Islamic culture where the acquisition of a given status is bound up with motherhood, together with that of a wife who works in the home performing functions which have become well defined by tradition. Both time and space have been distributed according to sex in a society where a binary view of social relations still predominates.

This panoply of differences or distances which applies clearly to a Franco–N.W. African couple is relevant, in part, to other couples where the difference in cultures and religions is less significant. Yet these distances do not exist in the same way in the case of people who have a different social status. Indeed geographic distance, for instance, can be significantly reduced if the couple have ample funds to enable them to travel freely. There is a significant difference between the embassy official living in Paris and the skilled worker from Berliet living in Lyon who 'has burnt his bridges' as far as his place of origin is concerned. Moreover, the solution to everyday problems may be eased if the partners have had a higher level of education so that they can formulate appropriate courses of action and express themselves articulately in dealings with government officials. The level of education will have a direct effect on the settlement of conflicts, and on the way the couples deal with their children. The fact, for example, that both partners are engaged in some profession may enable each of them to appreciate the other in his or her own cultural context. The inroads made by certain feminist ideas on roles and status within the relationship will be easier to take for a couple who are aware of developments, which they will be able to take at a certain intellectual level, than for a working class couple faced with a difficult existence. Thus a difference in a person's original social standing and his or her present lifestyle will, at times, outweigh such objective differences as place of birth, colour and language.

Distances are relative. Their intensity will vary from one couple to another, and will depend on time and place. What is regarded as 'mixed' here today, may not have been so yesterday in another country. A whole realm of perceptions of these differences will come into being through the subjective eyes of each partner, which in turn will have been conditioned by that person's level of social education and also by the nature of the bond which ties him or her to their original group and to the group of their partner. Moreover, a given difference may have been accepted by a couple, but will this be the case all the time, from time to time, or never again after a certain point? The ability to discuss these differences will create a mosaic of agreements, a marital consensus which may never be completely accepted. The acceptance of a difference passes through the conscious recognition of what it is in its own right and what it represents for the other person. Why, for example, does a Muslim partner, who does not in any way practise his or her religion, insist that their son be circumcised? To avoid and dismiss such questions will leave a misunderstanding hanging in the air, and this could reappear whenever a conflict arises. The place and role of the individual are different in each culture. But they are also determined by the circumstances in which one lives, by one's age, etc. The underlying requirement of each partner is in effect, above and beyond recognition of that person's individual identity, recognition of the identity of the group to which he or she belongs and of their community of origin.

'You cannot say you love me if you hate my people' (Man from N.W. Africa, aged 28).

These differences within a mixed couple are highlighted depending on the culture and nationality of origin. A Franco-German couple which now, thirty years after the end of the 1939–45 war, seems to have a problem-free marriage, especially if they are of the same religion, may still come up against differences at certain times. For instance, since qualifications in the two countries do not exactly coincide, this can lead to professional relegation. This is the case for a French nurse who is employed beneath the level of her qualifications which are not recognised in Germany. The French partner will have to adapt to a different daily pace and, among other things, eating more at breakfast to make up for a light lunch, followed by a more substantial dinner in the evening. There will also be a difference in the way meals are regarded, especially if the French partner has been used to traditional cooking, prepared that very day. A Franco-Swiss (or Franco-Belgian) couple will have fewer difficulties in adapting because they do not have any real sense of national boundaries if they live in a French-speaking canton. In the case of a Franco-Italian couple, on the other hand, if the foreign partner emigrated some years ago, references to Mediterranean culture may surface at certain times. Having the same religion and nationality does not cancel the real cultural differences between a couple where one partner is from France and the other from the French West Indies. The idea of the traditional family will make an appearance if the willingness of the other to admit certain differences is not forthcoming. It will appear like the return of a repressed social identity—the return 'of the socially repressed person'.

'I had never seen him in that state' (French woman married to a West Indian).

This has to do with a new discovery about her husband who, having drunk a few glasses of rum, started to dance in public in a way she would never have thought him capable of: 'He was almost in a trance and dancing very strangely'. She now has a different way of regarding her husband whom she had thought to be quite normal if not competely gallicised.

Is it not alcohol which has caused the divorce of a Franco-British couple in which the French wife was unable to accept her husband's regular visits to the pub? This may be an accepted social custom in Great Britain, but it was looked down on by the social class to which this French woman belonged.

We see another example in Tunis where Belgian women married to Tunisians suddenly feel an urge to be back 'among Belgians'. Like the German women who, in 1972, set up the 'Association of German Women Married to Foreigners', on the initiative of Rosi Wolf Almanasreh, married to a Jordanian and living in Frankfurt. According to the West German bulletin *Sozial-Report* (1979), more than forty contact centres have been set up around West Germany. The consciousness of differences between married partners has led these women to create a suitable structure of their own.

Many Polish women married to Frenchmen and who have lived in France for a number of years, even if they do not express the wish to stand out from the French culture that they have assimilated, will nevertheless feel the need for a religious observance which amazes their French husbands.

Let us not forget that it has taken decades of persistent ecumenical effort to reduce the enormous distances in France between the Catholics and the Protestants, despite the fact they share the same culture. These distances are still just as real in Ireland.

An Armenian married to a French woman, who has been living in France for forty years, suddenly reveals a hidden identity to his wife and tries to introduce a return to his roots by a visit to Armenia. Then he starts listening to Armenian music. Nothing like this has ever happened in their marriage before.

Does not the resurgence of anti-semitism bring about signs of a resurgence of Jewish identity and of religious practices? Since she thought her husband was fully integrated into the culture, the French wife is surprised that he wants the child she is expecting to be given a Jewish name.

Another French woman, of Muslim background, the daughter of a harki, now a Catholic of many years standing, surprises her husband by her ever more frequent visits to her family and by her sudden decision to keep Ramadan, as a visible, tangible sign of belonging to her original community, the one from which her parents were transplanted.

In the same way a Romany gypsy will suddenly leave his office job, which he had obtained with difficulty after taking a professional training course. He now plans to buy a caravan and to live like the 'travelling folk'.

The partners in a Judeo-Christian couple whom I met in Pittsburgh (Pennsylvania) in July 1980, went completely separate ways when it came to choosing the new President of the United States. The man, who is pragmatic and decisive, voted for Reagan, because he had had enough, at sixty years of age, of seeing America 'going down hill as the whole world looks on', whereas his wife, a Jewish emigree from Hungary, was unable to vote for a candidate who, in her opinion, held demagogic and dangerous views. After thirty-five years of marriage, during which time they had always voted for the same candidate, she voted for Jimmy Carter.

Indeed, partners in a mixed couple know right from the start that objective differences exist, but they have not always appreciated how significant these differences might become at certain moments. They will resurface, at certain periods, with the same force with which they were buried or camouflaged. Couples will very soon come to realise this truth.

Is this not the lesson they can teach couples in which the partners are not mixed? Indeed, in a mixed couple, the partners are alerted to possible conflict. They must bear this in mind and endeavour to overcome it. To some extent, this can lead them to become more aware of one another's needs. They will try to get to grips with certain unforeseeables which could spoil their marriage relationship. They know that, at least on certain points, they are different from one another. In a non-mixed couple, on the other hand, the partners may have no idea that there could be anything to separate them. The (supposedly) almost complete convergence of their views and outlook causes them to be unaware of the real differences that exist or that might one day exist. A clear understanding of the situation may then be too late. After several years of married life, the harshness of a crisis may be fatal. The partners are disarmed, they often have neither the time nor the energy to reconsider their marriage.

In the mixed couple the distances are quickly recognised at the start of married life, or through a complex web of small crises. Through these conflicts a minimum consensus of opinion will form — though this will never be rigid — and this may well serve to avoid a fatal crisis later on. *This slight advance notice is one chance the mixed couple has.* Firstly, it makes it possible to quickly identify significant differences; and secondly, it enables them to create a stable way of living together which caters for the existence of each partner.

The mixed couple which gives in at the first crisis is heading for an early divorce. However, in their youth and in the intense compelling nature of their love relationship they may find the resources to overcome these great difficulties. The *desire* to create a marriage will not be eroded as in non-mixed marriages where the *partners*, well matched superficially, sometimes believe themselves quite capable of overcoming anything that might try to separate them at various times in the future. They have not foreseen the possibility of a fatal breakdown in this apparent agreement and understanding they have. In the mixed marriage, on the other hand, the stark reality of the sum of the differences between them, guides the partners, through situations of real tension, towards a progressive cultural attitude and outlook. They are not so ill prepared. They know in advance what may happen. Alerted to the problems they may encounter in their partner, each of them is able to be more aware of the other.

Beyond all the problems we have identified, and their varying levels of intensity, frequency and ambivalence, there is at stake a greater recognition of the personality of one's partner as a separate individual, identified by his or her uniqueness and desires. This journey of mutual recognition is not completed overnight. The compelling relationship of the first romantic encounter, which is thought so much of, will not in itself achieve anything. At this stage, the partners are living as lovers before they have got to know one another. When the mask of romanticism and novelty is dropped they will find themselves, through the development of a loving maturity, as husband and wife, and as the mother and father of children. With time, their identities will re-establish their original foundations, those handed down to them by their original social environments. Each is then surprised by the other as they turn out to be different from the people they seemed to be when they fell in love. It is here that we see the importance of communication with one's partner in order to understand things that come to light, things one had never been aware of before. 'He is, after all, quite different, and yet he is himself; I too am different. Will he recognise me?' They may no longer be recognisable on certain points, but have they maintained sufficient contact in their communication with one another? One still needs to know how to communicate when one has to recognise the other as a Stranger. Nevertheless, communication in a mixed couple will be no straightforward affair. Their words will surprise them and put their relationship to the test. Words here become traps, rather than ways of becoming free together. We also need to consider non-verbal communication . . .

# 6 Intercultural communication

*'What do you mean when you say ...'*

*'Love what I am deep down inside and not what you want me to be superficially'.*

This statement caused a sudden hush among friends at a dinner party. It was not taken from an Ingmar Bergmann film. It shows us very clearly the need people have to be recognised. 'You must recognise me where I am most likely to be truly recognised', the man continued in the quiet which followed. Without noticing his talent for literary creation and research, his wife was continually reproaching him in public because he showed no interest in do-it-yourself. He could no longer put up with being forced to please her in an area in which he knew he had least chance of succeeding. He would use the following metaphor to express how he saw the situation: 'If only my wife would recognise me for who I am in my own field where I know what harvest I am capable of producing!' Though a legitimate need, this recognition is, at the same time, difficult to achieve in an absolute sense.

Mixed marriage is very representative of couples in which the relationship is defined by needs. The many expectations and desires make it essential that dialogue between the partners be true communication.

'A good marriage consists of a blind wife and a deaf husband', said Montaigne.[1] Leaving aside the usual interpretation of this, it may be that this sixteenth century French writer also meant that the partners knew one another so well, they did not need to look and listen. Mixed marriage is certainly at variance with this ambiguous statement. What Montaigne probably meant is that nothing should be taken for granted in a relationship; the blind need to learn to see and the deaf to speak.

This total dialogue is achieved in words and through sexuality. It is not obvious; on the contrary, it is beset with traps and with the circumstances of everyday life. How can one actually interpret what is taking place between a couple if one fails to take into account their past, their social status, and their personal experience of life? How is the desire for the other person to be expressed and received? Dialogue between the partners must find its own structure in terms of the relationship the couple have. Communication is certainly one important, tangible aspect of the couple's life. The quality of this communication will depend partly on the desire to reach the other person, and partly on the ability to express oneself. Words and gestures can produce stormy exchanges. It is rather the way they are channelled which will give these exchanges the quality of 'things communicated'!

'I've adapted more to you than you have to me' (American song). How can one ensure that communication between partners is a reciprocal exchange and not just the adaptation and alignment of one with the other, in other words resignation?

John W., a Briton of Welsh descent, can never understand why his French wife always says to him, before friends, when they are taking aperitifs: 'You English with your Guinness . . .' In this she is expressing the whole social relationship of cultural differences between French and British customs. In the first place, it is not really the done thing to drink beer as an aperitif in France; and in the second place, this drink which is so popular with the British, has become very important to her Welsh husband in light of his expatriation. Apart from the fact that the wife's remark has the effect of minimising this aspect, it also expresses a woman's attitude (not at all as positive as the male view) to beer in general. This same John W. also says: 'I find it much easier to have a row with an Englishman than with a Frenchman, despite my many years of learning the language'.

In a mixed couple the partners face the risk of placing too much importance on this immediacy of response and on the stark reactions of the other, which may surprise and shock them. At the same time partners tend to underestimate both the elaborate process by which this spontaneity is produced and the technique necessary for this type of intercultural communication. There is no guarantee at all that one will understand the other by his or her reactions, since these are a manifestation encoded by their cultures. Lengthy training in decoding these messages is therefore required. In the mixed couple, much more so than in the non-mixed couple, and especially if the partners do not have the same mother tongue, the difference in the spoken word (and, as we shall see, in what is communicated in gestures) is the concrete translation of a social reality which is perceived in different ways.

She told me about Ramadan and I told her about Lent. Later I discovered that they weren't quite the same (Frenchman, aged 28).

He had in mind the ascetic, Christian fast, strongly inspired by the Gospels, with connotations of penitence and the idea of withdrawing from the world into an internal desert. He had failed to understand the social festive function of the fast in Islam. Ramadan is an occasion for re-establishing one's Muslim identity. Although recognised, this practice is somewhat twisted and looked down on in Europe, as for example in the French slang expression 'faire du ramdam', meaning 'to make a din'. This is far removed from the mystical function assigned to it by Al Ghazzali (Muslim thinker, died 1111).

The other person cannot be perceived as someone who has been truly identified if his speech, gestures, habits and the general posture and movement of his or her body have not been properly recognised and interpreted in the light of their culture. People need to be recognised both individually and as a member of a cultural group from which they have been temporarily removed. A Muslim man will not be able to stand his French wife saying to him that he is 'not like other people'. He feels as though his cultural origins are being seriously denied. She is trying to isolate him from his own group, cutting him off from his roots. 'Not to recognise me for who I am is to require that I go unnoticed. Is she ashamed of me? Then why did she marry me?' Thus, in the dialogue between the partners in this marriage there will be a number of needs and requirements at several levels: there will be the level of true discourse, and the level of the need to have one's identity recognised as an independent personality not divorced from its culture. In the non-mixed couple, too, the partners will require this same recognition, though with less intensity because they are from the same country and have the same language. The fact that one of the partners in a mixed marriage will feel, to some extent, an exile, will influence this demand for recognition in dialogue.

It will be essential, in light of the daily efforts at communication by the partners, disjointed because of their different cultures, that cultural decoding takes place. How important does one's partner see religion? How, for instance, should *she* interpret the fact that he avoids certain foods, if *he* is a Jew or a Muslim, since *he* does not practise his religion in any other way? Or the fact that he insists on their son being circumcised? Furthermore, differences of class culture have a part to play here. It is likely (as borne out in experience) that a partner's ability to assimilate the culture of the other will depend on their level of education. The Senegalese lawyer, married to a French woman, will have certain advantages in the same situation over his compatriot, who is a skilled worker, which will enable him to appreciate certain cultural subtleties. He will see a number of benefits in his partner's culture. The reason is that he will be decoding what he experiences, not only on the basis of his own culture, but on the basis of his social position.

The way a person lives, walks, sleeps and washes are all expressions of his or her original and present culture and social position. Are their ties to religion of an intellectual and cerebral nature, or are they at the practical daily or seasonal (festivals and ceremonies) level? What are the factors and influences that have structured and continue to structure the individual as a cultural subject? Is his or her concept of the separation and distinction between the religious, the secular, the neutral, the political, and between the sacred and the profane, clear-cut? Where are the boundaries, and have they always been placed in those positions? If a partner's thinking has been structured by a very different culture, there will be whole areas in which ambiguities, incomprehensions and conflicts can arise.

The religious understanding may be quite harmonious between a Protestant man and a Catholic woman in whom a common culture has instilled a sense of agreement. They will readily come to an understanding on the religious education of their children. They will also be helped in this by recent moves arising out of the teaching on active ecumenism. But will the same thing apply for a broad French Catholic married to a Madagascan Protestant?

One couple aged fifty and married for twenty years, in which the husband is Italian, struck a balance over the religious education of their two children. Their common Catholic religion did not divide them, but the rural religious expression of the husband, a native of the Abruzzi region, has sometimes exasperated his wife: 'Oh, all that's only superstition . . .'

A Jewish woman begins to resent more and more the fact that she is married to a Christian, feeling that her group identity has been cast aside. She is now faced with the question of her son's religious affiliation. Her husband cannot understand this because he no longer thought of her as Jewish and felt that she had accepted the lifestyle of his Catholic family since she had been willing to marry in church. Although they are political militants of the left, they do not have quite the same point of view on racism and anti-semitism . . . Fundamental differences of opinion on Israel, Zionism and Palestine begin to create serious rifts in their relationship.

Misunderstandings arise in a Franco-German couple in connection with views on meals: the French husband is used to traditional cooking, whereas his wife is not prepared to devote the time required. In addition to the division of tasks between the man and woman in a marriage, we see here two opposing cultural views. After several years of life together, they have to come to terms with something which is separating them. Every individual is modelled, from early childhood, by his family environment which, in turn, forms part of a larger cultural group. His or her personality is formed by all this cultural and social heritage. The individual becomes, to some extent, a product of a cultural difference which asserts itself when faced with another culture.

Just as two partners from the same country and from the same background will, through various mental mechanisms, instantly and naturally decode what they see and hear in their relationship, so the mixed couple will have to carry out a systematic decoding of the culture of each partner. One partner will have to act as interpreter of the other's actions, words and gestures. This daily interpretation will be essential if they want to find common ground. Otherwise areas of ambiguity will remain in their relationships and these may result in endless misunderstandings and conflicts. The search for common ground here will come about through the forging of bonds which did not exist at the start. Neither partner married the other stripped of any context; they were, at the same time, marrying into a culture and a past of which the individual is simply a concrete expression, but a complete, concentrated expression. The individual, this strange partner, is a part which expresses the totality of a multitude of socio-cultural areas whose roots are buried in the collective memory.

Indeed, each partner is required to get to know the other's world, perhaps to learn the other's language if they really want to understand the other's personality. Regular dialogue is an act which requires a great deal of good will on each side. As well as being one another's translators, they are also one another's interpreters. If they do not share the same mother tongue, their verbal communication will come up against barriers which they may be able to push back by some other form of communication, supplementing their words with gestures.

Particularly in its sexual and erotic expression, gesture takes the place of speech. What is actually happening in simple verbal communication and in the use of the mother tongue of one of the partners? This is the situation facing couples who speak different native languages as, for example, in a Franco-American couple. The French wife speaks one or more sounds, i.e. words in her own language, thinking of the overall sense she wants to convey. Her American husband hears sounds which he identifies in French and must then mentally translate at once in order for them to have any meaning for him. But the sense which his translation gives to those sounds is not always the one his French partner wanted to convey.

The first time she asked me to go and buy a 'bâtard' [bastard; mongrel; type of loaf], I thought she was pulling my leg. I thought it was just a joke!' (American, aged 35).

His wife, born and brought up in Paris, had failed to realise, in the full flow of conversation, that the term 'bâtard', for an American who had recently arrived in France, did not mean a sort of loaf, but that it was taken in its literal sense of a child whose father was unknown or, even more widely, a person one does not think very much of, in common slang. The difference in meaning here is important, especially since this word is not used with the same meaning all over France.

Dialogue within a mixed couple will move towards irreducible fixed terms between the partners. Areas of understanding and shorthand expressions will be adopted on the basis of these fixed terms. They will become superfluous insofar as it is no longer absolutely essential for them to speak in order to make themselves understood. They will have acquired and, in certain areas, built up together, a common language, free from misunderstandings. In this type of couple — more than in the case of a couple that shares the same language — communication is truly a matter of practice: it is not so much a question of the speech and language of each partner; rather it is something which, in addition to words, includes situations and even silence. How is one to interpret the communication which makes use of silence, unless by the fact that the word 'silence' has different connotations for different cultures? This view of communication involves thought, attention and reaction to the other person. It may be utopian or a luxury for some couples, or in some situations, for the often utilitarian, abrupt aspect of discussions between partners does not allow for the quality of dialogue which will enable communication to take place. Moreover situations crop up which had not been foreseen and which escape the most watchful eye. The partners then react instantly, often in trying circumstances, and this acts as a breeding ground for conflicts. Linguistic misunderstandings are often born out of unforeseen difficulties, that is to say, situations one could not have foreseen.

The examples of communication situations in the mixed couple can help to unravel the complexity of dialogue in all couples. Taking a Franco-N.W. African couple as an example, since they demonstrate the characteristic differences (culture, religion, language), let us try to identify the importance of what is at stake for the partners in such a marriage. This type of couple is quite frequently encountered in France in certain suburbs of large industrial towns where N.W. African immigrants have tended to grow in numbers over the decades. This particular couple lives in a provincial town. The husband, from a rural background, completely illiterate in French and Arabic, has been in France for twenty years. He has been back to Algeria twice with his three children, all of whom have Muslim forenames. He has kept his Algerian nationality. His wife was divorced; her first husband, a Frenchman, provides maintenance for their two children. Originally from the working class, she has basic educational qualifications. She takes care of all the paperwork in the marriage. In order to avoid interference in their affairs by the authorities, and to make it somewhat easier for their children to become fully integrated into French society, they were married after many years of living together. The children now have French nationality. The wife does not know Arabic, her husband's first language. They met at a dance in 1957.

This couple faces a communication problem as the result of a disagreement with a gendarme following a car accident. The husband, speaking to his wife, uses the phrase 'your boliceman' [sic]; she replies: 'That was a gendarme, not a boliceman, as you put it'. Not only is she in a position of power as regards the linguistic relationship within the couple (since he is illiterate, he has not gained an adequate command of the French language), she also finds it hard to understand his difficulty in pronouncing certain French sounds which do not exist, or which are interchangeable, in Arabic. His words show a confusion between the sounds b and p, the latter of which does not exist in Arabic. Moreover, the confusion between gendarme and policeman indicates that he has not grasped the difference between these two functions in the French system. Lastly, he is confronting his French wife with the police image of her society, of which he as a foreigner — rightly or wrongly — feels himself to be a victim.

In a second situation, we find him listening to Arab music. She asks him to switch off the radio, claiming that the children do not like that sort of music. The prohibition is extended to the whole family. This is enough to make the husband go off into another room with his transistor and isolate himself. Here he feels a double resentment about his exile. 'It's important for me to listen to Radio Algiers in the evening', he says. 'But you should understand that Radio Algiers doesn't have a lot of meaning for us', she replies. It seems impossible to share some things. If she made an effort to listen to his music she would think she was wasting her time: 'With all this work to do, I haven't even got time to listen to my favourite record, what do you expect . . .' A difference of tastes, accentuated by the social conditions of life for this working class family for whom leisure time is given over to amusement rather than to learning something and taking an interest in another person's culture.

Unravelling the third communication problem of this couple sheds light on the wife's emotional subjectivity. Watching a television report on a bloody Palestinian raid, she exclaims indignantly: 'How obscene'. She expects him to express his agreement, and immediately interprets his silence: 'You think they're right then, since you aren't saying anything'. Being an Arab, he is unable to fully condemn this act of Palestinian violence which is in response to an earlier Israeli raid. He nevertheless has political opinions which are more in favour of a settlement of the hostilities, taking account of certain Israeli territorial positions. But what is actually the issue here is the nature of silence itself on the part of the husband. She interprets it as assent, harking back to the generalisation of the proverb: 'he who says nothing, consents', whereas silence in his culture can mean waiting time, time to reflect and meditate. His wife has never been to Bou-Saada, the Algerian oasis, where he spent all his childhood. She cannot fully understand the nature of this silence which can be a rampart against offensive aggression, rather than the expression of passive isolation. To stop speaking and express no opinion at once is not, for him, an expression of disagreement; it may simply indicate the need to think before speaking. This waiting time is immediately filled by his partner who reacts violently with a hasty judgment.

Thus daily communication can be the cause of countless ambiguities and even conflicts to varying extents. The will to understand the other person is not enough. It needs to be accompanied by an overall detailed study of the mental structures of the culture in question. If the partner simply takes words at their face value, that is to say if he or she makes no effort to decode the message and identify the possible different meanings, there will be no understanding nor being understood.

Even more enlightening is an analysis of the fourth communication situation. 'My wife . . . she takes care of the paperwork', he says. To which his wife retorts: 'She . . . she does have a name . . . I'm fed up always being referred to as "she" when you're talking about me'. The wife launches a bitter attack against her husband for using the third person singular pronoun when speaking about her in a conversation. She cannot stand it . . .Her husband is using a grammatical construction which requires a pronoun to support a noun. In French, this construction is rarely used and is considered sloppy. The French wife feels offended, as though the pronoun introduced a pejorative or dismissive element of contempt into what was being said. In Arabic, this construction is quite normal: the subject noun is very often echoed by a pronoun, usually in the third person singular or plural. This device of speech can actually be encountered in some popular French expressions.[2] This incorrect use of language shows that the foreign partner speaks French with the syntactical, i.e. the mental, structures of the Arabic language. He does not so much speak French as a type of French, while thinking in Arabic. His wife, on the other hand, thinks, understands and speaks French.

These linguistic misunderstandings, if they are never explained, will result in incomprehension due simply to an incorrect interpretation arising out of a lack of, let us say, grammatical and linguistic competence. Each speech conveys a certain number of facts and they produce a certain number of reactions in the partner. In this couple the linguistic power ratio is uneven: not only is the Algerian husband unable to speak his own language to those closest to him — his wife and his children — he is also unable to express himself correctly in their language, which results in a number of misunderstandings. This situation of inequality places the foreign partner in an inferior position in the marriage, as well as in the whole family's social relations with society at large. This situation leaves the whole linguistic field for the French partner to take care of.

'You speak; you're the one who knows how'.

He thus recognises her competence to speak in his place before other people and quite correctly acknowledges her monopoly. She therefore has linguistic power both in and outside of their relationship as well as the ability to exercise it alone. Her husband will therefore feel obliged to allow her to manage their children in terms of any dealings they need to have with public bodies. Language here is an exchangeable currency. To a certain extent he will be excluded from this round of exchanges since he does not have the right currency. Or, to put it another way, he has a language which is not quite legal tender in the transactions in question, like old bank notes or coins that are no longer valid. It will fall to her, in this family, to discuss matters with teachers, social security and welfare workers, officials and neighbours. She has no need to keep as close a watch on her speech as he would have to, running the risk of making mistakes. If by chance or by design he is involved in such matters, his contributions are likely to be clumsy. He will be afraid that he lacks the necessary arguments. She, again, is the one who is most able to stand up for the family and for the children. He is excluded from the area of speech, excluded from taking part in a whole linguistic system which is the medium through which a whole range of important matters is dealt with.

A study of the above four situations shows quite clearly his difficulty in understanding and in making himself understood.

'At best, dialogue between them can only take this form!'

The reason for this is that there is no conscious awareness of the existence of a code. The woman merely resorts to attacking her husband when she cannot understand him. The two partners see their respective cultures as opposed to one another. They lack all the necessary socio-cultural skills to understand differences and to decode one another's behaviour. Inequality here takes the form of social and cultural inequality. They are unable to deal with situations of conflict in their conversation, not only at the level of their reactions and emotions, but also at the level of cultural decoding. In a Franco-N.W. African couple of the professional classes, the same situations, having been perceived at the first level, would have been decoded or interpreted differently at the second level. There would of course be considerable differences in that mastery of the French language by a N.W. African doctor would mean that he never confused the sounds *b* and *p*. The reactions could be similar in the third situation (the Palestinian raid), however, because the emotional aspect can so easily override a rational attitude which would require a great deal of self-control from the wife just in order to control her indignation. This control is not always possible, particularly at the time when such emotions are exchanged.

Similar situations to these, in which lack of understanding is highlighted, are also encountered in French couples. The partners in a working class couple have similar codes against the background of the same mother tongue, and common points of reference for understanding one another, even if a husband from the Vendée region uses certain dialect terms when talking to his Alsatian wife. But she will understand despite his regional dialect which may only be a matter of accent. In our example of the Franco-N.W. African couple, on the other hand, the lack of understanding in the four situations is aggravated by the fact that their original cultures are different. The partners have each been differently programmed, both from a social and an ethnic point of view. They will not be able to enjoy a level of communication which can remove these conflicts.

In the case of a Franco-Spanish couple in which the wife is from Lille, and in which both partners were office workers in Biarritz, communication was not without its misunderstanding at the start of their marriage. They have agreed to base their life together in Spain, however, since she no longer has any family in the north. She has been well received into her husband's family and has accepted certain family codes. Her integration has also resulted in her taking a Spanish course and she now speaks the language well.

I now realise the enormous benefit in being able to speak my husband's language. I can also understand the mistakes he is likely to make when speaking French (French woman, aged 30).

This couple made an effort, right at the start of their relationship, to reduce the linguistic barrier. Indeed, in this case the French partner was attracted by Spanish culture and she is now quite at home with it. This is a true conversion: in marrying her husband, she also married Spain. But her personal social and family situation may also have had a part to play in her integration. She 'did not have a great deal to lose' leaving the north of France where she no longer had any emotional ties. She was, to an extent without roots. 'She had everything to gain' in her new attachment.

In many mixed couples their conversation is just not on the same wavelength if neither partner will come out of his or her linguistic isolation. Should such great stress be placed on spoken language? To reach perfection in this area of understanding will never be possible. To wish that the other partner speak exactly the same language is perhaps to refuse that person the right to be foreign, as well as not recognising another way of seeing and appreciating situations.

I did however manage to get him to stop saying hamdu-llah[3] at the end of meals (French woman employee, married to a Moroccan official).

This woman is preventing her husband from expressing a phrase which has religious connotations at the end of a meal. At one and the same time, using general secular, Cartesian logic, she is preventing herself from understanding the deep significance, not only of the expression her husband is always uttering, but also of the role that meals play for the Muslim. She has not yet deciphered the full hidden meaning of her husband's culture. She only has a partial understanding of who he is: she is actually 'ordering' him to integrate and to become like the French. She is requiring that he fall into line with the cultural norms of the French. By exerting pressure on him, she is undermining the points of reference which mark out his identity. This deprivation could have serious consequences and lead to psychological disturbances.[4]

For this skilled Moroccan worker, expressing certain words meant re-establishing his identity. If this is to be denied him, it could serve to heighten his anxiety. On the other hand, and the distinction is important, a more sophisticated N.W. African will have the necessary resources for evaluating situations and will be sensitive to not uttering such expressions in certain circumstances. In the light of his wife's disapproval, an Englishman, married to a French woman, stopped drinking beer at certain times at his wife's insistence. Then one day he made a fool of himself at a dinner party by drinking far too much, which led to a dramatic confrontation. 'I told you, it's actually in their blood', his wife exclaimed to her friends.

**Notes to Chapter 6**

1. *Essays*, Book III, Chapter V.
2. In Le *Langage Populaire* [Popular Speech] by H. Bauche, Paris: Payot, 1951, we read, on page 131: 'Le charretier, il bat ses bourrins' ['The carter, he whips his horses'].
3. In Islam, 'Hamdu-llah' is an expression which means 'Praise to Allah'. It is quite often uttered to thank God for some good thing.
4. In a very commendable book, *La Plus Haute des Solitudes* [The Greatest Solitude], Paris: Seuil, 1978, Tahar Ben Jelloun described the problems experienced by immigrant workers in France.

# 7 Body and sexuality

*'I heard a lot about black people'*

Dialogue does not consist purely of the confusion of mannerisms and expressions. It also involves sharing and accepting explanations: 'Giving pleasure to the other person, so long as it is not always unpleasant for oneself'. The English concept of feedback is very important and indeed necessary for communication within a mixed marriage. It not only implies a certain reciprocity, but also a certain technique in that reciprocity. As we said earlier, transparent dialogue in a life shared with a foreigner is not at all straightforward. It requires discussion and explanations. The 'meta-linguistic' function, as defined by R. Jacobson[1], holds a privileged position among all the functions of language. It is this which makes provision for the necessary reassessments and calm explanations in order to come up with a broader marital understanding. A true consensus of opinion between the partners will form the basis of their relationship. It does not of course cancel the differences between them, but recognises and identifies them. One's partner is made to face up to another voice, other words, other means of expression, and other ways of thinking. This confrontation should not result in the abdication of one of the partners, but in his or her recognition. A true dialectic relationship is established between husband and wife and this makes it possible for them to reach joint agreement. This couple, far from becoming a shapeless whole ('one flesh') in its thinking, where one partner subjects the other in terms of words, speech, ways of looking at things, instead becomes an harmonious duet, two points of view which are brought together, sometimes achieving a consensus, revealing something that was not evident before. Situations of constraint can change moods, feelings and anger into violent, degrading arguments.

> We noticed that we were often inclined to hurt one another when we were having money problems. Both he and I are on edge at times like that (French woman teacher, married to a Briton).

> On some occasions, in this same couple, the husband took it badly

when his wife refused his sexual overtures. There were evasive attitudes and manoeuvres. What was being communicated at such times was the denial of a certain power in the partner. In a relationship with another person one's mode of speech alters and adopts patterns either as an expression of drawing closer together or as an indication of distance and moving apart. The coming together in dialogue, in the first encounter, is characteristic. Words tend to create closeness. In this first surprise of happy encounter the lovers are launching out into the unknown in order to find pleasure together. They will want to be like each other, adopting identical behaviour, matching the tone of their voices and their speech rhythms. This extends to the pauses which punctuate the verbal interaction, when the lovers share a silence which draws them together. The intensity of this mutual, uniting discourse runs the risk of losing its force as the partners get to know one another more after the initial surprise of encounter. Elements of difference and even disassociation start to appear in this relationship which at first was so close. Perhaps also, depending on the situation, the partners show a desire for areas of demarcation between them so as not to lose their individual identities. Wanting to find themselves 'completely in the other', the merging of their lives has led to a confusion in which they can no longer recognise themselves.

Jean did not speak French very well. In the West Indies they learn French at school, but speak Creole amongst themselves. He sometimes makes remarks in Creole and speaks it with his friends. He has covered up most of his West Indian personality in order to become 'French'. I, on the other hand, having lived in the West Indies for a while, have now come back to earth and am becoming reintegrated into my own 'environment' (French woman, aged 28, two children).

This young woman shows quite clearly how, for her part, she has returned to the French identity which she had more or less suppressed at the start of the relationship with her West Indian partner. The initial alignment is now giving way to the search for a balance in their relationship: 'We eat both French and West Indian style. We listen to West Indian music'. But what from her point of view appears as a return to her identity and reintegration into her own environment, is seen by her partner as as kind of 'renunciation'. In this case, the importance of the living environment and the presence of two small children has led them to seek a *modus vivendi* which is not just a false harmony in which 'everything is in everything'. Since her husband cannot competely master a language which is not his mother tongue, he sometimes expresses himself in Creole. By this he is demonstrating his West Indian origin in the context of a French identity which he is trying to acquire.

But he knows he will never acquire it fully because of his physical characteristics and the colour of his skin. Nevertheless his West Indian identity is French for legal purposes. He is French like the rest, but with a special West Indian element; he is trying to acquire a predominantly European French identity, like that of his partner. Deep down inside, he knows he will never accomplish this and that it will be too costly a depersonalisation for him. He also knows that he is closer, on some points, to his West Indian friends with whom he shares the same skin colour, language and a whole series of mannerisms and traits which his wife will never be able to penetrate and fully understand. In this couple complete sharing will be difficult to achieve: 'I know when he stands at the window looking up at the sky that it is the sky of the West Indies he is thinking about'. She can only guess at this. She is aware that there are certain limits to what he is able to share. More than in the case of an ordinary couple, the partners in a mixed marriage will realise that they cannot share everything and that at certain moments, one's partner becomes withdrawn as he re-enters his first solitude.

He has his world and I have mine. There are some things I cannot understand, and there are likewise things that he cannot understand (French woman, aged 40, married to a foreigner for 15 years).

In another Franco-American couple living in a small town in central France where they have been for two years following a lengthy period in various states in the U.S.A. after their marriage fifteen years ago, complete mastery of the English language by the French wife has made it possible for her to adapt her language to various situations.

'We speak English between ourselves, but mostly French to the children' (French woman, aged 36, married to an American).

In this marriage, daily use of the foreign husband's mother tongue produces a balance in their communication and a presence of the other person's culture. On the other hand, the use of French to the children, who were born in California and spent several years there, also equalises the influence of each language, particularly in a completely French environment. The American here has an advantage over the West Indian partner we looked at above whose wife did not speak Creole.

In communication between a mixed couple, therefore, we see a number of elements which have to do with the use of language. We have seen how, in some couples, there can be continual misunderstandings and disagreements when one partner has failed to appreciate the workings of the linguistic system which has shaped the other partner's way of thinking.

If one partner is unable to translate, this can lead to difficulties in understanding. Indeed the mere fact of understanding one another's words does not mean that one is making oneself understood. The need, at certain points, to pass beyond the words can be a barrier between the partners in a relationship. To a certain extent one needs to forget the words and retain only their sense. A foreign language is used as an instrument which one has not always learned to use properly. Words, in fact, only communicate part of the message one wants to get across to the other person. Perhaps there is some truth in Maurice Blanchot's statement that 'all direct communication (using language) is impossible'.[2]

It certainly comes up against various barriers for mixed couples as well as for non-mixed couples. However, to try to reduce this effect by words alone would be too restrictive. The partners will find in their sexuality a language which is communicated with the body. The whole invisible area of verbal communication will be assisted (not to say enriched) by this body communication in which the silent yet meaningful phrases of touch and gesture are uttered. Words are a reference to that part of the brain's activity over which an individual has a different level of command. But here too, in the language of the body, we will find contradictions, areas of opposition, limitations, false assumptions and ambiguities, as with verbal communication. Moreover, it is impossible to make an arbitrary distinction between verbal communication and body communication because sexuality is also expressed in words! To what extent will the physical communication of the couple's bodies also reflect the state of communication that exists between them in their relationship as a whole?

A mixed couple's sexuality is not confined to physical body-to-body contact between the partners. The body can enhance the emotional life of the relationship in general. It is used alongside verbal communication. It is not meant to be excluded. It is an essential visual cue for one's partner: the body is the medium for facial expressions, gestures, movements, as well as of warmth and impressions. Smiles, looks, caresses are expressions that can go beyond the limitations of words which, at times, can be inadequate to express subtle feelings connected with the desire to give and to accept. The body is essential not only for one's partner, but also for oneself. Is it not the case that to love oneself is the starting point for being able to love another person? In their sexuality the mixed couple will employ many variations. Discovery of the other will be an unmitigated surprise.

I had heard a lot about the sexuality of black people so it took me a long time to get rid of certain ideas. The first time I touched a black hand, I felt that I was truly different. I was gaining access to another continent. All that, of course, was my imagination, merely fantasy. But that didn't prevent it from being an emotional discovery (French woman, aged 25, student).

Whilst expressing this attraction, she also spoke of the great fear and, above all, the feeling of guilt to begin with in terms of her own social group. Moreover, this young woman shows a tendency to place too high a value on her experience, which was a new one for her. She immersed herself in her fantasy in order to derive pleasure from the encounter:

I was aware that I was taking great risks. Having been attracted, I let myself go. I didn't stop to think; deep down inside I knew that this great pleasure I was allowing myself was breaking the rules.

She was actually separating herself from her close family, her friends and from her whole social environment in going out with a black African. The physical attraction was a real one.

The sexual relationship is a clear indication of the extreme limits which groups set up to mark out their boundaries. The contact between groups can have to do with economics, trade or war. It is these relations which bring them together as groups and societies. But the sexual relationship is a 'line of demarcation' which it is difficult for individuals to cross because it strikes at the heart of the social group on which its future depends, the reproduction of the group as a whole. The sexual relationship is one link in the reproduction chain. It is for this reason that it is always monitored in all societies, sometimes in the form of strict rules (particularly in terms of virginity for young women), but also in family systems where the choice of marriage partner is more or less imposed from outside. In some cultures, the individual is not entirely free to choose his or her partner: it is the social group that directs the partners in their choice. Marriage is more a social act than a private one. Even in so-called liberal western societies there are a large number of relationships, including sexual ones, which are brought to an end just before the couple becomes engaged . . . Marriage becomes the regulator of sexuality, particularly with regard to the consequences which might arise. C. Levi-Strauss describes this:

Social recognition of marriage, that is to say, the transformation of the sexual encounter based on promiscuity into a contract, ceremony or sacrament, is always a difficult adventure, so we can see why society has sought to protect itself against the risks involved by the continual and almost neurotic imposition of its mark.[3]

A foreign individual who 'touches' one member of a group introduces something different, and this is sometimes seen as a 'pollution' of the group in the eyes of the members as a whole. This is why mixed marriages have not only been disapproved of — and still are in some cultures, religions or ethnic groups — but are also forbidden. All these social prohibitions have tended to feed the imagination of individuals so that sexual relations have become a taboo subject between them. For the very reason that it is taboo, it is seen by some people as attractive and exciting.

'This time it's different' (French woman, aged 30).

The area of the forbidden is one in which the imagination can be very fertile, both for social groups as a whole and for the unassuming individual in his or her everyday life. A whole series of ready-made judgments, or prejudices, with respect to blacks, Arabs and Jews is drawn from views which have been inherited from one's culture and from history. These have an effect, consciously or unconsciously, on the relationship between two foreign individuals:

> When I first started going out with Philippe my uncle told me that I was lucky! Because I would be very satisfied at the sexual level, more so than with a Frenchman (French woman living with a black African).

Since they do not marry like other people, or at least like the majority of people, and 'are looking for something different, which extends to the area of sex', this marriage which differs from the social norm cannot be like ordinary marriages in terms of sexuality! The partners have set themselves apart and live in a different way. It is in this context that negative value judgments and curiosity arise.

It is again C. Levi-Strauss who points out the relationship between the taboo of incest and that of mixed marriage in that the latter is a type of exogamous marriage which societies have not been able to codify in a satisfactory way. Thus the distant partner is proscribed, as are relations with one's father, mother, brothers and sisters. This fear of things that are too close or too distant would seem to form part of the same principle. What is at stake is preservation of the group identity.

Erotic literature has played its part in feeding these fantasies, particularly in connection with the foreign woman. If she is Swedish, she will be a blonde. If she is Asian, she will be a small long-haired brunette. If she is black, she will be seen as a 'Negress' brimming with sexuality and not as puritanic as the white woman who has been brought up in a Christian culture. At the same time she is threatening, dangerous, and even perhaps bordering on a deviant type of sexuality. She will satisfy perverse desires. If she is Italian, she will be warm and plump. If she is a Muslim, she will be fat and inextricably linked with the harem. There are a whole host of images to feed these sexual fantasies. The same thing goes for the man, whether he be black, Arab, Jew, Nordic, etc. The unknown is forbidden and the forbidden partner quickly becomes the focus for an imaginary sexuality. The other person becomes an inexhaustible source of all sorts of fantasies.

I must admit, I can understand women wanting to go to bed with blacks, but I can't understand those who want to get involved with Arabs (Frenchman in the street, November 1978).

In his book *La Rumeur d'Orléans* [The Clamour of Orleans][4], Edgar Morin presents a scenario of a whole world of threatening fantasies. This book, based on research carried out in the city of Orleans, shows how Jewish traders were able to be involved in the white slave trade. The Jew is thus a threat, sexually, for the non-Jewish group. In the same way as blacks are seen as a threat by the whites of the Southern States.

But this threat is not mutual or equal for the two sexes. Whereas wanting to go to bed with a black man is seen by the social group in an unfavourable light, wanting to go to bed with a black woman (a 'Negress') is seen as a sign of virility and as an exploit . . . provided the individual concerned only looks on the relationship as a physical, non-emotional one and that there is no intention to marry the woman. 'Hm, she looks very nice; very tempting!' said a twenty-three year old Frenchman looking at a black model in a fashion show on French television. Thus each separate individual lives in a world of fantasies of their own, and these may go as far as latent perverse tendencies which a foreigner is able to reveal.

The partners in a mixed marriage will to some extent be influenced by all these collective impressions, these ideas of what other people are like. Their sexual relationship will therefore be found in a world which is sometimes difficult to understand in abstract terms. In some instances it may be distorted:

I was made to feel like a whore because I sleep with a West Indian man . . . but I don't just sleep with him, I live with him and have had two children with him (French woman, aged 28).

Society projects a debased image of the most intimate relationship between such partners. This is primarily racism, but it shows, at another level, that the group feels its identity is under attack. This negative (or indifferent) attitude is a defence mechanism which feeds on preconceived ideas. Thus a whole system of resistances and preconceived ideas surround, isolate and distance the outsider and confine him or her to a downgraded status. What develops is the required level of distancing in order to protect one's social group and its identity.

If he were my neighbour, I might be able to accept him. Though I'm not sure. But to become friends with him: no, I don't think I could do it. It is something stronger than myself (Frenchman, aged 32).

The marked distance here shows quite clearly the boundary that this man does not wish to cross, whereas for another person the relationship would go further, to the point of becoming a deep friendship, for instance. The person in question might still not be ready for 'his daughter to marry his best black friend', however. Whereas marriage in general is a structure for equal exchanges, mixed marriage, as C. Levi-Strauss says, is 'an unequal marriage'. And for the social group as a whole it is a 'bad marriage' onto which it will project negative ideas, attempting to justify them by stressing everything (particularly in the area of sexual fantasy) which enables it to identify the foreigner with an uncodified (if not corrupt) exercise of sexuality. It will in this way justify its racism and try to substantiate its attitude in expressions showing an aversion for the outsider. The Lebanese are difficult; you can never get away from them. Blacks are villains because of their colour. The white Arab is a 'stinker'[5] (this is an indirect reference to filth and dirtiness; thus he smells!).

Confrontation in a crisis is not only related to a marriage situation; it is also a cultural thing. Verbal communication and sexuality are a reference to the body of the other person as the habitation of an intimate identity. They bear a direct relationship to this system of differences and distances which one has chosen to accept in return for certain compensating factors. But what differences or distance is a partner really able to accept in the other? Is it really accepted? And to what extent? For how long? Is this difference expressed in unusual ways, acceptable at certain times, or is it a permanent, daily grind in the details of life at close quarters with another person?

I had to accept a lot of small things: the way he ate, his culture, his pace of life, the way he washed. It was a long time, for instance, before I understood the way in which a N.W. African washed his face. One day, when we were on a trip together to his village, I saw the men performing their ritual ablutions in the street, washing with a very small amount of water and no flannel. They rub their faces like this with their bare hands. So it was not until several years after we had got married that I saw this link with the way my husband acts, something I had never been able to fully understand or been able to accept. I had made a value judgment about the way he washed. What at the start of our relationship was something new for me, and something which gave me a pleasurable excitement, 'this something never experienced before', has of course become blunted over the years. The initial difference becomes difficult to live with day in day out (French woman, aged 32).

This woman was able to attribute a significant content to her husband's actions when she had the chance of seeing them in their context. Once they have been accepted, they can even be valued in an emotionally mature relationship, even though the initial novelty has worn off. Communication in the couple becomes the effect of a long apprenticeship. Each partner perceives the other through the eyes of his or her own mother tongue. Will they speak the same language?

Even though we speak the same language, we are not on the same wavelength (Frenchman, aged 42).

The same words had different meanings and so did the silences:

My wife cannot understand my need for silence at certain times (N.W. African, aged 35).

Moreover, she cannot understand him if she refuses to try to understand the meaning of this attitude:

It is just like a wall. Once in bed, he is very active; but I need to be prepared with words before we make love. He doesn't. I feel as though I am just a sexual object whose only purpose is to give pleasure. This creates many problems between us (French woman, aged 33, married to the above N.W. African).

Silence on the part of her husband is interpreted by this woman as non-communication and even as an attack on her personality. The man is unable to understand why she refuses him this right of silence. She has never been to her husband's country and is therefore incapable of understanding all that silence means for him. Even less can she appreciate the social and rural significance of this environment. Was he really neglecting talking to his wife? He had conversations, throughout the day, with his colleagues ... Moreover, he did not see the connection his wife made between talking to one another and making love.

There are many non-mixed couples who experience exactly the same thing, though they do not necessarily seize on sexuality as the area in which the differences lie. They will tend rather to look first for reasons in one another's psychological make-up. The mixed couple cannot explain everything away by *psychological* reasoning. Far more likely will they be led to look for *sociological* reasons for their differences. Is this awareness of all these aspects to the life of a couple a luxury, a choice or a necessity? These perceptions are quite clearly affected by the social and cultural position of the couple and of each of the partners. But they do not suppress sudden emotions, blunders and acute crises.

'I can't stand his smell any more with his Arab habits' (French woman, aged 40).

This sudden value judgment is expressed in a crisis which shows a marked trace of marital racism, a sort of slip on the part of a socially and intimately suppressed person. Although until this point all available defences had been employed to counter this expression of racism, it now returns, like a boomerang, in all its stark reality, causing the partner pain and injury. The other person actually has a real *and* symbolic smell, classified in a sort of olfactory hierarchy. Smell in itself has a social status of great significance. The above exasperated remark by the wife is a crystallisation of the contempt she has felt for some time, which may surprise even her. Her remark provokes a somewhat violent response from her husband:

She was always saying: you should take a shower, never noticing the times when I did wash. She was always checking up. I realised that she was unable to accept my body odour . . . Yes that's it, she couldn't stand my smell (N.W. African, aged 40).

Does this bring us up against distances which cannot be reduced or shortened for some people, except at a great price? The other person's smell affects us in our subconscious at a level we have not yet perhaps discovered or want to discover, so hidden we are afraid to admit it. The other person's smell thus acts as a threat, because of its power. It is a reminder of the social group and of the original identity. Although it is well camouflaged by all those deodorants and sophisticated perfumes which indicate the desire to merge with the identity of the prevailing social group, this smell of the other person acts as a reminder of the time when he or she lived quite differently in another country. It acts as a trigger for deeply hidden messages. The person on the receiving end interprets it in a 'good' or a 'bad' light, depending on their own past experience. It directly addresses one's intimate experiences. Smell is then able to produce an approving, welcoming response, or feelings of revulsion and aversion.

It is a physical thing; I just can't explain it. I can never get into a taxi that is being driven by a black man, because of the smell. It's something I just can't explain (French woman, aged 50).

Smells that disgust, or smells that excite and arouse. It is reminiscent of those tourists who have been to Sicily and then speak about the smell of the peasant women they came into contact with. Real *and* symbolic, smell thus has a practical effect on one's judgment of the other person; and this is heightened if that judgment is based on the imaginary ideas evoked by a certain smell. The idea behind a smell can be stronger than the smell itself!

It is important for partners to discuss their sexuality. But this will depend on the dual relationship which they will tend to overvalue, just because it is at the edge of the social group. Dialogue is often not expressed in words alone. The human body is invested with different qualities depending on the culture and on the social classes. It will to a greater or lesser degree be the place for the imagination and for desire, the primary forum for exchange, and this includes exchanges of the imagination and desires.

'I was fascinated by his black skin. I gave too great an importance to it' (French woman, aged 28).

At the same time as an awareness of breaking a taboo in entering into a relationship with an outsider, there is also a tendency towards an erotic overvaluation, and towards a carnal romanticism which would like to ignore all boundaries and limits:

'Making love to a woman who has shaved her pubis can be quite stimulating' (Frenchman, aged 50).

At the same time the other person's body takes on a very great importance: it becomes the place in which the foreign partner, the exile, can take root and assimilate the other person's past. It is the body-territory, the place of imagination and possession. It reminds the foreign partner of his or her mother's body to which there was such an attachment that removal is a difficult experience, producing feelings of great jealousy or longing at the slightest absence.

Sexual freedom, and body freedom in general, will be a subject for lengthy discussion in a mixed couple. Depending on cultural origins and religion, there will be marked variations codifying conduct, the way in which one should dress and go out, and the individual attitudes of the group:

I just can't understand how the French can allow their women to expose their breasts on the beach. Something is destroyed by that sort of behaviour (Spaniard, aged 40).

This reaction to the phenomenon of nudity is not restricted to Mediterranean countries; it is also encountered in certain circles in France. The supposed sexual freedom of the Scandinavians is not always the case, nor is the exaggerated jealousy of the Mediterraneans or blacks. Here, too, preconceived ideas continue to have their effect.

Nevertheless, adultery with someone of the same type is very difficult to bear on the part of the foreign partner. It is seen as a direct threat, as though the guilty party were saying, contemptuously: 'You're only a foreigner'. Taken as an insult, it marks a distancing between the partners in a relationship in which the foreign partner had made a much greater investment than the love received in return. The foreign partner will feel betrayed, doubly exiled from his or her country and from the lost partner.

Moreover, this sexual freedom will often be judged negatively from the outside. It is an indication of something distorted in the couple's relationship: 'I could have told you it wouldn't last'. It is the search for the social implications that people will come back to at the slightest sign of trouble. This sexual freedom will often create problems for certain mixed couples in which the partners have made such a passionate commitment to one another just because, in light of the various forms of opposition they had to face, they could *count on one another's love*.

The passion they have created between them, right at the heart of their relationship as a couple, through their feelings, thoughts and, perhaps, an overflowing sensuality — just because of its taboo nature — may now be too demanding, and perhaps even possessive and exclusive. The attempt by one partner to become less dependent may not be interpreted as a desire for greater freedom, but as an attack which is difficult to bear:

I just couldn't accept it. I sacrificed everything for him: my family, my country. Although I didn't become a Muslim myself, I accepted the fact that my children were Muslim. And then he goes off with a young woman from his own country. I just don't know what to do. My children are the only reason for living I have left. I feel lost. It is difficult to admit. It seems as though I am not the mother of these children, nor his wife. I am being made to suffer the devaluation of my own body, and I will need to face it in solitude and at the beginning of old age (French woman, aged 45).

Immersed in bitterness and pain, this woman feels devastated by the extra-marital affair of her husband who now wants to calm her down. He tells her that it does not mean anything. His idea of sexuality is different from hers. The situation is identical for a non-mixed couple, but here it is seen in a more dramatic light. The wife, an exile from her own country of birth, is unable to stand back and minimise her situation. Is she not surrounded by younger competitors who are also more like him? Having first experienced the attraction and fascination for someone different from his own people, he is now feeling the same attraction for people like himself. Is he not going back to his original identity? Will he not be even more different afterwards, more faithful to himself?

In their communication, therefore, the partners are unable to 'expel' their deeply rooted differences. Differences also resurface in a Franco-Japanese couple. She went to live in Tokyo with her Japanese husband, a company executive. It was a great surprise for her to discover how boys and girls in Japan are educated and brought up separately. It is not surprising that her husband would sometimes appear savagely virile, expecting her to be extremely feminine! She realised how much this could affect both the level of communication between her and her husband, and their sex life. At times he insisted that she fit in with the stereotype of the Japanese woman!

A woman should be submissive and discreet, she should not indulge in mockery, she should love her mother-in-law and serve her husband, she should never interfere in important matters . . .

This quote from a famous book,[6] sums up the principles of femininity. Not that women are seen as representatives of weakness because they have great power, in particular the family budget and upbringing of the children, with importance equivalent to that of the mother-in-law. A certain reserve is expected from them in their attitudes and in their conversation. At the sexual level great change is taking place and reality no longer corresponds to what Ruth Benedict wrote: 'Sex is an area in which the Japanese do not moralise as we do. Sex, for them, as in the case of all other human feelings, is good in its own place, and that place is a minor one in life'.[7] The exasperation of desire expressed in the film *L'Empire des Sens* [Empire of the Senses] is an extreme example, because the status of sexuality is changing in Japan along with the development of marriage for love. The words 'I love you' in Japanese, mean 'I want/desire you'.

If the words do not have the same meaning from one culture to another, the exercise of sexuality is also subject to variations which will require adaptation on the part of the partners in a relationship . . . But is it not precisely this fascination with the unknown which some people are seeking?

His voice has a very sexual quality to it. Sometimes he sings and I like that very much. It is quite the opposite of the Deller Consort singing. The castrato voice doesn't do anything for me (French woman, aged 25).

This woman is very fond of her boy-friend's strong, deep, sexy, male voice, which resembles that of her father. His strong, warm voice adds to her feeling of sexual enjoyment. The fantasy finds a concrete expression, rather like those soothing women's voices on the radio which encourage 'an emotional regression to a state in which one is again captive to one's mother's voice'.[8]

Sexuality and communication within a mixed couple, as we have seen, require cultural translation and this must take place in real-life situations. Words and gestures define the identity of one's partner in a reciprocal exchange. Hesitation, refusal and doubt alternate with unconditional longing and desire for the other person. It is also a search for one's own identity, not completely free from ambiguity.

> She wants him to want her
> He wants her to want him
>
> To get him to want her
>  she pretends she wants him
>
> To get her to want him
>  he pretends he wants her

| Jack wants | Jill wants |
|---|---|
| Jill's want of Jack | Jack's want of Jill |
| so | so |
| Jack tells Jill | Jill tells Jack |
| Jack wants Jill | Jill wants Jack |

a perfect contract[9]

## Notes to Chapter 7

1. 'Closing statements: Linguistics and poetry', in T. A. Sebok (ed.), *Style in Language*. New York, 1960.
2. *Faux-Pas*, Paris: NRF, 1943, pp. 21 and 30.

3.  *Les Structures de la Parenté* [The Structures of Kinship], 2nd edition. Paris: La
    Haye Monton, pp. 650–651.
4.  Le Seuil, Paris 1969.
5.  Cf. Augustin Barbara, *Mariages Mixtes* [Mixed Marriages], Thesis presented
    to the EHESS (the College for Higher Studies in Social Sciences), Paris 1978,
    400 pp. plus appendices.
6.  Kaibara Ekiken (1790).
7.  *Le Chrysanthème et le Sabre* [The Chrysanthemum and the Sabre], Chapter 9.
8.  Mr. Bernard, 'La strategie orale ou la transvocalisation' [Oral strategy or
    transvocalisation], *Esprit*, No. 43–44, July-August 1980, p. 57.
9.  In R.D. Laing, *Noeuds* [Knots]. Paris: Stock. 1977, p. 10.

# 8 Specific marital practices

*'I sense a certain curiosity from people'*

At the start of their life together the partners in a mixed couple are reticent to acknowledge any special aspects to their relationship:

'There is no difference between us and other couples' (Chilean, aged 35).

This desire not to stand out from others often leads mixed couples to the point of wanting to dismiss even the most obvious aspects of their mixed relationship. This alignment with other couples may be carried to an extreme:

I had always thought that he was French and fully integrated into the French way of life. Then suddenly he starts talking more and more about Vietnam (French woman, aged 42, married to a Vietnamese).

Because she wanted their marriage to be completely 'like the others', this woman has always thought of her husband as being like other French people. She has not always noticed how difficult it was for him to integrate and the questions in his mind: 'Vietnam no longer exists, he's never had any news'. She has forgotten his country and family too quickly. She thought that with their two children, she and her husband had somehow forgotten all about Vietnam. The matter was not settled in his mind, however. More and more this man's native land gains in importance for him, although his ties have long since been severed. He is now engaged in receiving Asian refugees and is on the committee which organises the annual festival activities. He starts welcoming his compatriots into his home; this upsets his wife who sees her home becoming more and more Vietnamese. The children also find it difficult to come to terms with this aspect of their father's personality, having thought of him as being French like everyone else. The partners start noticing differences which separate them; they then notice differences which distinguish them from other couples. Moreover all their efforts at alignment will eventually come up against certain limits, because a mixed couple is open to the most critical judgment from society at large. The mixed aspects of their relationship, which they wanted to dismiss as unimportant, will be brought back to their attention on various occasions. By marrying a foreigner, a member of a group has succeeded in 'standing out' from the rest. The couple will therefore be the object of 'social marking'.

His wife is Jewish and practices her religion. What's more, their children don't have Christian forenames (Secretary, aged 30).

The work colleague of this man who is a manager in a large private company, sees herself implicitly as the spokesperson for the opinion of the social group. One cannot deny the factual truth of what she says, but it is the social aspects she is alluding to. She communicates it in terms of objective differences: the Jewish religion of the man's wife. But there are here a number of expressions which show the distances these two individuals have covered in order to move away from the centre of the group and end up on its periphery:

'She couldn't marry a Frenchman like everyone else'.

'They haven't even had the children baptised.'

'He's French, of course, but he's also West Indian.'

'Because no one round her wanted her, she had to settle for this black man.'

'He was rather weird, that chap; always seemed distant in a strange sort of way. It doesn't surprise me that he married a foreigner and became a Muslim.'

It would seem that the mixed couple's efforts to establish an identity are more successful on an individual level than on the social level. After all, the individual has turned his or her back on the group, preferring to sort things out alone. This distancing of oneself from the group is something their families recognise to varying degrees. In a way — as the above expressions show — this marriage ostensibly turns its back on the group, on the way it operates, and on its rules. Having set themselves apart, the individuals will look for all possible reasons to justify their unusual, or even incomprehensible behaviour to the group in general. Indeed, by their escape they are affecting not only the identity of the group but also a whole series of interrelated factors. Moreover, they may act as an example to other members of the group who will dare to imitate them. They have highlighted a loophole of escape; their marriage has become a sort of safe haven. They are acting alone, for their individual benefit and not for that of the group. This first reaction may indeed evolve so that new relations are established which will make room for a new dialogue. The reason for this is that, depending on who the partner is, the group may derive some secondary benefit from the union. In this case, the individual success of one member also involves a degree of social success for the group as a whole.

A young woman from the country, who has studied for a few years and who, through her marriage to an older African student on his way up the government ladder in his own country, becomes the wife of an influential minister, gives her social group cause for pride in the promotion acquired by this differing type of lateral marriage. Although the members of the group may have disapproved of her running away, they will now derive a certain advantage from her marriage when, visiting her in her adopted land, they find themselves given a royal welcome.

In the same way an individual disadvantage can to an extent become a social disadvantage when the member who moves away from the centre of the group no longer feels a bond with what had been his or her natural environment or roots. The individual concerned is in some way placing himself on the outside. It also represents a disadvantage for the group in that it did not have the necessary resources to keep and integrate that individual. He has gone far away because the group did not hold sufficient attraction for him either now or for the future. In such cases the group will tend not to speak about the person's leaving as they would have done in the previous case where a certain amount of success had been achieved.

Because their plans take them outside of their groups, the partners in a mixed couple will feel unusual and different from other couples. Will they therefore be aware that they do not actually live quite like other couples?

The markedly different nature of their daily practices will be 'stamped' in accordance with how mixed a lifestyle they have, both within their relationship and in relation to other couples, and in accordance with the degree to which they fall into line culturally with the model for couples as determined by the dominant society in which they live. It is likely that a Franco-N.W. African couple in which both partners are from the working classes, living on a predominantly N.W. African council estate, will more often than not conform to the lifestyle of the latter, especially if the family lives nearby. It will adopt the same way of life, the same festivals and perhaps the same diet. Their children will relate to the children of immigrant workers and will feel close to them. In the same way, a couple in which the partners are international officials will have a lifestyle more in keeping with an upper class environment and may have greater opportunity of determining their own mixed practices. A working class couple will offer less resistance than the other to pressure to conform to the dominant standard. Moreover, a desire for isolation, or simply a wish to keep oneself to oneself, may lead the couple to develop mixed practices. These will have to do with religion, language, place of residence, cooking, etc. Will a Judeo-Christian family celebrate Christmas without resigning itself to making certain concessions to the in-laws? A Franco-Malaysian couple tries to reach a solution with regard to holidays: 'Every two years or so my wife goes to Malaysia to spend some time with her family. Unfortunately, we can't all go together, especially now that our family is growing.'[1]

This man, a doctor of science, is searching for a degree of balance in his family and is able to achieve this in part thanks to the financial resources he and his wife have. But he is aware that the possibilities are being eroded as the number of children they have increases (they have just had a third); these possibilities become less and less as one goes further down the social scale:

At the moment we are living from day to day. We once went to Martinique for a month (French woman, aged 28, living with a man from Martinique).

A single one-month trip in five years is not enough for this young woman to get a very clear idea of the country her partner comes from. She does however remember the unhappy impression she received of their 'chauvinism and the way men there take it for granted that they are entitled to be waited on hand and foot'. The trip enables her to see the reason for some of her partner's attitudes: 'I now realise what an effort he has to make'. From now on her feminism adopts a new approach. This couple is clearly at a disadvantage from the financial point of view. As a qualified secretary she provides a more regular source of income for their home than her partner who is a skilled worker without a permanent job. Because of his low salary, he feels inferior in terms of social status, and this is aggravated by his 'natural West Indian chauvinism' which makes it difficult for him to cope with this situation. Under these circumstances, holidays in Martinique will be very rare with two children to take into account. The family budget will not stretch that far.

In the case of a Franco-American couple, on the other hand, in which the husband is a commercial director and the wife a French school teacher, none of these difficulties exist:

'We live in France, but we both feel the American influence; we feel like tourists in France. We've only been back here two years'.

The situation is quite different and more favourable for this man and woman who, having met in the U.S.A., married and lived there for twelve years. Not only is there the factor of their socio-professional status, they also have more possibilities open to them than the Franco-West Indian couple referred to above. Moreover the age difference also explains a certain independence, a stabilisation of the family situation and the possibility of carrying out their own plans. Every other year they go for a holiday in the United States; they even have plans to return there for good . . . but with the option of returning to France if they find it difficult. The double insulation of ten years in age and social status enables a couple to practise a mixed lifestyle, whereas this is not possible for another couple, apart from the fact that a black West Indian, an unqualified skilled worker, will inevitably find it more difficult to integrate than a qualified white American. The Franco-American couple have the means to plan out their lives (allowing for the risks that involves) which the other younger couple do not.

## The Marriage Ceremony

Mixed practices do not only affect the choice of holidays; they become an issue on many occasions. They may already have played a part in the marriage ceremony. Indeed, whether it be civil or religious, the marriage ceremony often takes place in one partner's country in the almost total absence of the foreign partner's family. Moreover, if the two families are present at the ceremony, the coming together of two different cultural worlds can be a delicate one. The partners then become the intermediaries between the two families in order to introduce them to one another. Theirs will have been an important role in choosing the venue, menu, orchestra, and style of proceedings (elaborate or otherwise) . . . Most often, however, the foreign partner, particularly if from a very distant country, will find themselves at the wedding ceremony with only one or two members of their own family; indeed they may often be alone. All they will then have will be some close friends for support.

Although they met in the most romantic of circumstances (on a beach in the Vendée), Kassim and Violaine are typical representatives of the Muslim-Christian marriage. The decision to get married is sometimes accompanied by a firm resolve not to bring Islam and Christianity into conflict and even to be the instruments of an encounter which goes beyond the simple ecumenism of circumstances. This young Tunisian, an ordinary worker, is taking a social training course. His parents are of modest means. Violaine works in an office and has been deeply affected by her involvement with the MRJC (Rural Christian Youth Movement). Her parents have a small farm in a village south of the Loire and they have several children.

Kassim and Violaine both wanted a ceremony which would point to the drawing together of their two religions. Kassim is the only one present from his family (his parents were unable to come), but there are five fellow Muslims, alongside his bride's family and the large number of friends they have in common, both from the MRJC and from the MRAP (the Movement against Racism and for the Friendship of Peoples). The procession sets out on foot from the brides's home to the church where the ceremony will take place in the presence of five priests. The Muslim friends read texts from the Koran and another Muslim–Christian couple bear public witness to their own life together, highlighting the opportunity this union offers for being two different people and of discovering two cultures. In another ceremony, the foreign partner only has one friend of his own nationality to represent his community of origin. But the remoteness of the country of one partner does not always explain the at times marked (and significant) absence of the family.

We were married in Kansas City in 1965. The ceremony took place in a Unitarian church (an intellectual church where one does not pray). My husband's family was present and so was mine, apart from my parents. It was a grand wedding: about three hundred guests. Everyone approved. We lived in an international environment. We were in love and have had a very dynamic marriage.

The remoteness here is easily compensated for by the social status of the partners who were able to stage a grand celebration. It took the form of a grandiose justification. Roland Barthes says that 'a grand wedding is a response to the ancestral, exotic concept of nuptial celebration'.[2] Wedding ceremonies are an index of the level of acceptance or rejection on the part of the families and of the social groups involved. If they have been rejected by their families, the partners will tend to invite their friends, thereby creating a circle of social recognition which doubles for and replaces the absent family circle. Because the ceremony cannot be fully celebrated with their families, the couple looks for 'another family', their friends. If they have been more or less excluded from the family circle, they will feel obliged to form around them a circle of people who are in agreement with their plans.

'She's fully entitled to marry who she wants to, even if her parents don't like it' (a friend).

The wedding ceremony will highlight any disagreement between the families, as well as showing the solidarity of their friends. However, friends are less involved than families: they are not so directly affected by this marriage. They are only 'temporary, interim, or should we say replacement parents', in contrast with the real parents and family who have a living consciousness of their social group.

Marriage does of course take account of the groups to which the partners belong, and it is for this reason that it is not an improvised affair. The choice of a wedding date will not only take into account the availability of close and distant relations, but also of social commitments. In the rural areas of France, weddings have always tended to take place outside of periods of intense activity. Similarly, weddings on the coast of Brittany and on the islands only used to take place after the fishing season and depending on how fruitful the catch had been. In addition to this, the church did not allow weddings at certain times (Advent, Lent). Even in towns today, weddings are far more likely to take place on certain days and in certain months.

The celebration of mixed marriages does not always take account of these implied rules. Back at the wedding invitation stage we see the intention of affirming the 'sublime love of two individuals', rather than a sharing between two groups. The following announcement of a Muslim–Christian marriage appeared in 1978:

'There is always a path of discovery,
an opportunity to be seized,
a light somewhere,
a land to love . . .
We are pleased to invite you
to celebrate our Love
and to witness our mutual commitment . . .'

When the social groups are implicitly in agreement, they will not need to be 'converted' to this love. The celebration becomes a normal, natural and social recognition of the union. The groups are not social witnesses and this is not required of them. In the case of mixed marriage, it often happens that only one of the groups is involved because the other group is far away or culturally inaccessible. They cannot therefore begin to form social bonds to reinforce the marital bond between the partners. Often the bride rejects the traditional long wedding gown and chooses a light, 'new-look' dress, thus creating harmony between her dress and the unusual nature of the wedding. The bridal procession too, which is meant to be a demonstration of a precise, hierarchical order in the community, is often thrown off balance by a mixed marriage. It is necessary to look for substitutes: for example, a distant aunt will take the part of the mother of the bridegroom since there is no other representative of his family present.

To a certain extent, the celebration of this marriage reflects the lack of balance it will create in the social group. Sometimes, it is celebrated without any announcements; indeed in some cases the wedding announcements are sent out a few days afterwards, simply stating that 'X and Y were married quietly in Dakar'. Only the bride's father had gone to be with his daughter on her wedding day, a wedding celebrated with moving restraint 'in the presence of a handful of friends she had made there'.

Very often, not only do the couple marry against the wishes of their respective groups, but these groups are also hostile towards one another ... The ceremony then becomes a somewhat censured social act. Only with time can it become an approved private act. There will be an officially clandestine nature to the relationship which develops little by little. Thus, right at the public beginning to their married life, the partners will feel somewhat different to other couples:

'My wedding was nothing like that of my cousin who married a local boy'.

The wedding ceremony of the cousin brought together two families who knew each other, in the very village where they had been born and lived no more than a hundred yards apart. In addition to this, the ceremony was conducted by the family priest who had taken the couple through the catechism classes. Here we have an equal exchange in contrast with the unequal exchange produced by a mixed marriage.

Being different from other couples, the new marriage partners will then either hide or flaunt this difference. There is the practice of the double name. One only has to look at the letter boxes or visiting cards of these mixed couples.

Because our name ends in 'ni', we are often taken for Italians or Corsicans. That produces less racism than if people realise right away that it is a Moroccan name (French woman, married to a N.W. African).

The name one bears becomes a description, an excuse for social categorisation. And when this name is very distinct, it is borne with discretion so as not to arouse unwanted comments. There is a certain wish to go unnoticed:

'I don't really want to shout from the rooftops that my husband is a Muslim'.

This attitude is in sharp contrast with that adopted, as a challenge, by some couples. They judge that they are in any case categorised by society. They therefore tackle the problem head-on and anticipate the generally reticent attitude of those around them. However, attitudes to names can vary depending on times and nationalities. An Anglo-Saxon name may even be added as a sign of social distinction, whereas a German name has for a long time given rise to suspicions and questions such as: 'What's the origin of your name?' One couple had lived for more than a year in a flat, exchanging polite greetings with the other young neighbours, until one day when they had been invited in for drinks, they learned that the other occupants thought they were Jewish! Just because of their Franco-German name on the letter box: 'We've often wondered whether you were . . .'

## Cooking and Lifestyle

The place of residence will determine the domination of one language over the other. For people who start their married life in the U.S.A., English will have been the language for daily communication. But now that the couple in question lives in France, the American husband quietly starts speaking French. The reading of newspapers from his home country, especially when important events such as elections are taking place, takes up a considerable chunk of this man's leisure time; he also listens frequently to American radio. Within his marriage he reserves time to live out his American personality. During the course of the day he will listen to the repetitive American music of Philip Glass, although he knows this is not really his wife's sort of music: she did not get beyond Gershwin and West Side Story.

'Sometimes we eat Madagascan food; but we also eat Asian, North African, Italian and Spanish style' (Frenchman, aged 30, married to a Madagascan woman).

'Our daily life is no different to that of other couples — apart from the fact that we eat both French and American food' (French woman, aged 30, married to an American).

Whether it be in the area of domestic chores, living space, cooking, use of time, etc., the mixed couple will find itself in situations where the dividing up of such matters between the partners takes the form of a series of adjustments. These adjustments will come about in accordance with the dynamics of their relationship, but they will also be dependent on their environment. Because they live in France, a Congolese husband will go with his French wife to buy furniture from a local store. Depending on their budget, they will buy the same type of furniture as other French couples in the same social category and living in France. But in their home one will find reminders of Africa on the walls. Hangings and cloths will be hung up next to one or two musical instruments. There is a wooden xylophone as a symbol of Africa. The man plays these instruments to me with an attitude of concentration which speaks volumes about what he feels. Since he has been living in France with a French woman for many years now, he has adapted to the dominant cultural pattern, and the living space of this couple's home is played out in western style. As far as the purely material items are concerned, everything is functional and western. But Africa is nevertheless there, distantly, in a decorative, symbolic and musical guise.

In this sense this man is different from a great many black African workers who live in communities in the Paris area and build up functional structures which will guarantee them daily moments of African life. They regain their identity and make a clear distinction between their western working hours and the African time of their leisure activities, cooking and talking. This same Congolese man was obliged to give up his habit of taking a siesta. His work would not allow him this time for rest and recovery. Different concepts of time can affect some couples. On the one hand we have western time in which industrialisation has very quickly standardised, rarefied and streamlined periods so that 'time to oneself' is pigeonholed for the weekends and holidays. This efficient, clear-cut western time, neatly framed in agendas and timetables, has acquired a whole system of thinking based on profitability, rapid decision making and discussion which gets straight to the point. At the other extreme oriental time is based on cyclical thought patterns which allow space for feelings and discussion, which may never come to an obvious conclusion, but which result in well measured decisions once the words have run their natural course. This notion of time does not always make for an easy married life. When, for example, the husband never comes home from work at a regular time 'because he has met some of his compatriots in a café and spent a long time chatting with them about home'.

Nor is a mixed marriage quite like others when the African husband suddenly starts to do the cooking. Put off, to begin with, by a type of food she did not like, his wife is 'converted' to her husband's tastes after a few months and starts to cook African dishes herself, which her husband appreciates all the more for their spiciness. So whereas to begin with she was making him a concession by eating his cooking, she now gives him the gift of cooking for him what he likes. Does she not, for instance, accept the use of fingers when eating meat from chicken bones? She defends this habit in her husband when they are dining with friends where this freedom is not normally enjoyed. His in-laws quickly put him at ease: 'Don't feel embarrassed, just make yourself at home'. If this invitation is taken seriously, it means he can bypass the normal practice, in a small family circle which is aware of this everyday practice in certain parts of Africa, as well as in some social classes in Europe. 'He's actually enabled us to see meals in a new light; we do tend to make short work of them', says his mother-in-law!

Approval of various customs, habits, rituals, rules, morals and the culture of the other person does not come automatically. It depends on different levels of cultural confrontation. A mixed couple in which two intellectuals are brought together will perhaps find a harmonious way of life as a result of the (sometimes easier) mastery of certain situations. Not all mixed couples have this intellectual understanding, this necessary ability to stand back from a situation. This fair cultural sharing, this confrontation employing a proper exchange may be a luxury which some mixed marriage just cannot achieve.

Couples on a limited budget, for instance, will not always have the resources for sailing calmly through the state of mixed marriage. If, for example, they want to go on holiday to the foreign partner's country each year they will have to be economical in terms of leisure activities, a consideration which will not need to come into the thinking of two international officials who are married to one another. It is actually cultures which are in confrontation through two individuals who share the same space, the same time and the same desires, as well as the same constraints. Adherence, or unconditional 'conversion' to the culture of one's partner can only come about after several stages, in a subtle, complex system of concessions, needs, things surrendered by force of circumstance or imposed by the social environment, and constant adaptation. But the whole of this very sophisticated system of exchanges will be matched by an equally subtle system of compensations. 'I'll let you have this if you let me have that', the partners are constantly saying to one another unawares. We are, at the interpersonal level, in the realm of

thought which has to do with the gift and the 'counter-gift', as Marcel
Mauss puts it[3]. There are between husband and wife a whole range of
stratagems, including emotional ones, and various forms of exchange
which hide the precise rules by which they act on a day-to-day basis. All
these gifts, stamped with unselfishness in the couple's thinking, are
actually arrangements or accommodations at the dual level of very real
cultural confrontation between social groups.

As the place in which a system of concessions and services is in
operation, this marriage is also a place where the partners exchange not
only concrete things, but also a whole series of symbolic things which they
themselves may not always be aware of. In a Muslim–Christian couple,
living in a provincial area, the fact that the husband practices the fast of
Ramadan means that the whole family lives in a certain way for one month
of the year. This time can be a privileged one between the partners in
which they are able to show affectionate attention to one another and
explain to the children the meaning of this Muslin fast in comparison with
the Christian fast. In this same couple, the French wife, who is a
committed Catholic, joins in with her husband's fasting on some days. This
symbolic exchange between the partners will naturally lead them into a
deeper Islamic–Christian dialogue and to an attempt to create a circle of
other couples who share the same way of life. They will try to give their
children a religious education which will take account of both Islam and
Christianity. On certain occasions they pray as a family and their children
have been 'presented to God' in the presence of a community consisting
mainly of friends and in the presence of a priest who is an ardent advocate
for dialogue between Christians and Muslims. At certain points, however,
their religious practices are separate: she goes to church on Sundays;
sometimes he goes with her; he in turn has his own private religious
practices.

Thus the sharing of daily life in a mixed couple takes on a number
of different aspects and reaches to the most intimate parts of an
individual's personality. In this sense they feel themselves to be different
from other couples, not only in terms of the opinions they have about
themselves or the opinions other people may have about them, but also
in terms of the mixed practices they formulate together in a more or less
harmonious compromise.

## Intimate and External Identities

The image which a couple builds up of itself also takes into account how other people see them or how they imagine other people see them:

When we go out together, I sense a certain curiosity from people. This summer we went for a holiday in . . . When the owner of the house we were renting saw my husband get out of the car, he was taken aback and asked me if this was really my husband. He seemed very surprised.

A visible, physical distinguishing factor in one of the partners (skin colour, curly hair, pronounced accent, etc.) makes the couple aware of different levels of toleration: in some environments they are accepted, and in others they are not. But this difference does not always cross the barrier of the indifference they could wish for on certain occasions. To go unnoticed would be a sign of recognition, or of their integration into the cultural groups concerned. In this sense, how each partner relates to the difference in the other is experienced, perceived and dealt with differently. Without the ability to stand back, intellectually, a mixed black and white couple from the working classes will perhaps have an excessive awareness of how mixed they are, in contrast with an intellectual couple who will be able to stand back and take things in a more relaxed manner. The difference in social environment and level of education also has a part to play in this. The partners will therefore, by way of example, discount or choose those of their friends and relations who accept them as a mixed couple without in any way treating them differently because they are mixed or because of the visible or noticeable difference of one of the partners.

A mixed couple experiences its areas of difference internally as they come to terms with various aspects of the relationship, and it also experiences its intrinsic differences in relation to other people. The practices of daily life, in the majority of cases, are fairly similar to those of other couples, but there are some which differ. There is always a certain irreducible area in which the mixed nature of the relationship will affect certain aspects of the partners' lives. Even in the most assimilated and integrated of couples, there will be areas in which they are not altogether like most of the people around them. Everything will depend on the nature and importance of the difference which distinguishes them in the first instance. Another significant factor will be the degree to which they are willing to make an effort to become integrated or, in contrast, to stand out. Moreover, in the different circles of socialisation, and at different times, the majority group will have been able to establish relationships of acceptance, assimilation, absorption, naturalisation and standardisation, or, conversely, it may have established relations in which the couple is kept at a distance, ignored or actively rejected.

There is therefore a complex structure to this relationship between two people attempting to find a balance and a way of living together as a couple; there is also a complex structure of relationships between this couple and the outside world, that is to say society at large and the different groups of which it is formed and with which the couple will find itself in contact on a continuous basis or at certain times. This range of relationships both internal and external, will form a type of *mixed conjugality* which is not perhaps very different on the whole from other marriages, but which will on occasions stand out as decisions are made on the basis of the more important mixed aspects of the relationship. For example, Franco-German couples will clearly face the question of where they should live and they will tend to want to stay near to the border so as not to be far from either country. Being in close proximity to both countries will encourage them to keep close ties with both families, to divide up their holidays within the same year between the two sides of the border, and perhaps even to comtemplate going to a third country. This will be less the case for a Franco-American couple who will go on holiday to the country of the foreign partner. A Franco-N.W. African couple living in France — when they have the financial resources — will also tend to take a holiday in N.W. Africa.

> . . . We spend our holidays in Algeria; this enables M. and me to keep in touch with the family. Our daughter, Nadia, then enjoys a new sort of mixed experience which is not there for the rest of the year (French woman, aged 29).

These couples exhibit in various ways a whole range of lifestyles, combining two in order to produce a third lifestyle for the mixed couple. They will in this way develop strategies and patterns of behaviour in their dealings with others, and a whole code of conduct will develop internally for living as a mixed couple in the midst of non-mixed couples.

> 'As mixed couples we must show that it is possible to live in this way' (Muslim, aged 34).

Knowing they are different, and knowing that they are regarded as fragile because of this difference, the mixed couple will tend to think more deeply about their marriage than the non-mixed couple for whom, even if there is not the question of a mixed relationship, there will still be married life in general to consider. This *mixed condition* shows up some very important questions which the non-mixed couple often overlooks because they are not apparent. They are there all the same, even if not so intensely. The mixed couple will develop a mixed relationship which is both intimate and able to face the outside world. It is a sort of identity which they will exhibit all the more as they feel the eyes of other people on them. Having built up a certain status and identity the couple will affirm, justify and practise it. The greater the social visibility of a mixed couple in a given social environment, the more the couple will tend to place a high value on what at the start was regarded as a social handicap.

'Our marriage is more solid because it is attacked far more than other marriages . . .' (French woman, aged 29).

All this is unnecessary for a mixed couple taking a course at the Collège de France and who are able to go about unnoticed. They do not have to listen to remarks from their peers, simply because there is an intellectual tolerance, or even a form of self-control which prohibits the public expression of judgments which one might otherwise make. This couple will benefit from an intellectual regard or from the right to indifference, whereas a mixed couple from the working classes, marked by clear discriminating factors (skin colour, a foreign voice, religion) will be on the receiving end of such judgments the expression of which will not always be controlled, perhaps even verging on blatant racism.

On the basis of the image a couple has of itself, and the image(s) projected on it by outside groups to which the couple belong, comes into contact with or has nothing to do with at all, there will develop *a way of living together as a couple*, both an intimate type of relationship and an external type of relationship.

'I prefer my wife to answer the 'phone, because even here my voice gives me away' (black African, aged 35).

This couple has come to realise that they are identified as mixed even without being seen. After several years, they have come to an agreement between themselves, a sort of code of conduct with regard to the telephone. The husband has accepted the fact of never being first to answer the telephone if his wife is also there. In this way they avoid certain unkind thoughts and unpleasantness. His different sounding 'Negro' voice would not pass the filter of indifference. This was sometimes the cause of unpleasant allusions. In the light of this situation, the partners have modified their intimate relationship and come up with the consistent strategy of not revealing to strangers that they are a mixed couple, so as not to 'expose themselves more than they need to'.

The mixed couple lives in a context of intimacy which is dependent to a certain extent on the type of relations they have in external contexts: family groups, their working situations, leisure activities . . . The internal coherence or consistency of the couple will indeed depend on the nature and solidity of the bond between them, but it will also be dependent on their ability to resist any reactions, which may sometimes be aggressive, from their external environments. The more the partners are able to control this external environment, the more they will be able to manage the relationship between the two of them and to find appropriate bridges between themselves and other couples.

It is when one partner has a good knowledge of the other's language, of course, that he will be able to perceive a whole series of subtleties in the latter's world and the interests which dominate that world. If he is interested in Germanic authors, the French husband will be able to converse with his German wife on current trends in that literature. The French wife who is ignorant of the five pillars of Islam will be unable to talk with her husband about his religion, nor will she be able to appreciate the depth of the impression this has made on his childhood. Thus a whole aspect of the other's life will be excluded from the field of mutual awareness. Even at the social level and even within the same profession mixed marriage partners have to ask themselves what the other person is really like behind that profession, behind that social status. Behind identical practices in terms of work and leisure activities, etc., there is a symbolic universe which reinterprets everything else.

To a certain extent, agreement in all the areas of practice within the life of a couple may not be enough if one partner does not make an attempt to approach the symbolic world of the other. There is the level of everyday practice and the level of symbolism. One professional couple who had been students and had lived together for ten years, had explored very recess of the mixed nature of their relationship. The Muslim husband could not, however, conceal his difference. Although he was an atheist, he could not bring himself to eat pork. His wife understood his feelings: she only ate a little of it herself, and never in front of her husband. Their children also understood that on this point their father was 'unusual'.

The Muslim husband in this marriage had reached a very comfortable economic and social status, having climbed much further up the social ladder than many French people from the same social background as himself. He was known to have an undeniable professional competence, but there was in him some resistance which made him retain his original identity: he would never eat pork. By this symbolic gesture he showed that he belonged to the 'umma'[4] community of Muslims who respect this food taboo. Indeed, this was not the only indication of his original identity. A significant part of his leisure time was devoted to the reading of Arabic books. There were two identities within him: that of his social and economic status which was evidenced by his professional practices and his external relationships, and that of his private, intimate status to which only his wife and children had access. It is in this restricted, protected, loving environment that he was able to be himself without 'exposing' himself. He could live this double existence with a certain sense of balance. He had created for himself an inner territory which he inhabited at certain times and in which he could re-experience his private identity. In addition he was able to practice his social identity.

However, the extent to which a mixed couple bears its special or mixed nature as a handicap, something traumatic, a stigma[5] or indeed as an emblem, will consciously or unconsciously reinforce this image. A process of stigmatisation will develop in each couple, and in light of what G. Devereux says about identity and personality, the mixed couple may have a 'mixed personality' and may function — to a greater or lesser degree of adaptability — with a 'mixed identity'.[6] This identity is formed in relations with others. The 'close mixed marriage relationship' is distinguished from the 'close non-mixed marriage relationship'.

Confrontation causes differences to arise and this sometimes leads to an exaggerated distinction. The mixed nature of the relationship can then become grounds for 'exhibition', and for a very conscious affirmation of the relationship. Being mixed leads to living and acting in a mixed fashion. But this mixed personality can, quite unconsciously, be internalised and translated into unusual practices which separate the mixed couple from other couples. At certain moments and in certain areas, these practices have every reason to be special in order that they might show respect for the original identity of one of the partners.

Sometimes, however, they can also be 'forced', overvalued in order to make them look special. The mixed nature of the relationship then becomes a pretext for 'not being like everyone else', because it may be seen as a pleasant thing to feel that one is original or 'on the edge of things'. This is then a way of saying that being mixed is a more interesting way to live than not being mixed, or even of saying that being mixed offers a higher quality of life. By reinforcing itself, it acquires substance in the statements made about it in conversations with friends and strangers. It will also justify itself and 'over-legitimise' itself. At the same time it will also reinforce itself to the couple themselves. The partners will find a whole system of standards for living as a couple and as a family (with their children) both in the home and outside.

In the intracultural (non-mixed) and homogamous (in the same social environment) marriage, the partners start out, at least, having many points of agreement and the ways in which they live will already be quite close in terms of environment, language and religion. They may subsequently introduce practices into this united, uniform and undifferentiated domain which will distinguish them at certain times from one another and distinguish them, as a couple, from others. Any differences which they may introduce into their relationship will not be interpreted by others as being of any fundamental significance since they are already known to be in a state of equality.

In the mixed couple this is not the case. The partners will try to come up with special mixed practices of their own which will reinforce their relationship, the reason being that there were no historic roots to their relationship before their first encounter. The couple has a joint history of its own waiting to be written as they reach consensus about their lives together.

C. Levi-Strauss writes: 'The game thus appears disjunctive: it ends up in the creation of a differential gap between the individual players or teams for whom, at the outset, there was nothing to indicate any inequality'.[7] In this text he makes a distinction between games and rituals. Games create a gap between players or teams who are in principle equal and have the same power. It is disjunctive. Rituals, on the other hand, are conjunctive. They produce unity. Mixed practices become for the partners in a mixed marriage rituals which might also be called 'conjunctive'. It all depends on the importance, repetition and rhythm of the exercise of these rituals. These conjunctive and disjunctive aspects appear here as the two sides of a hill in the marital landscape. Whether it be in the intercultural (mixed) marriage or in the intracultural (simple) marriage, there develops between the partners a whole subtle set of games and rituals which tend in alternate phases to encourage conjunction or disjunction.

In the mixed couple a real *intercultural strategy* will guide the nature and intensity of these mixed practices (place of residence, the children's education, nationality, choice of professions). The couple will actually live its daily life conscious of the difference that exists, striving for a balance both at the marital level and at the social level (outside of the couple). It will alternate between the desire for a certain indifference and the desire for exhibition, display or even for further exposure. Indifference will be preferred at times when the mixed nature of the relationship attracts no benefits from outside. This will be the case for couples in working class environments who can derive no benefit from their difference. Any social exposure they engage in will only mean social 'marking'. Exhibition by an intellectual couple, on the other hand may produce an exposure from which they can derive a symbolic secondary benefit. It displays its mixed nature as something which distinguishes it and which may confer an original status on it from which some advantage may be derived. Difference here is more a differentiation which is allied to distinction.[8]

> Daily life makes me aware that we are not the 'classic couple', when we go out shopping together, for instance, or when we go out for whatever reason. I know that we are different from other couples even if it is only an external difference, perhaps because he is black and I am white (French woman, aged 31).

Each couple finds itself in a *classified way of living* of its own, shaped by mixed practices and by a *mixed condition* which places a certain value on its mixed nature. This mixed condition may at times mean nothing other than that one partner is black. In some cases a couple may feel itself to be categorised or labelled. Even if an intellectual takes no account of this fact, the social environment will remind him of it on various occasions. In the case of a novel writer or essayist, living with a West Indian woman may be an unconscious symbolic plus in the aura of possibilities he allows himself in the symbolic area of permitted values. His social environment will accept it as something to be valued or as a permitted luxury, though not something to which anyone is entitled. The couple is not called into question. On the contrary, it is seen as a marriage of aesthetes. Originality here is added to the career of a famous author, intellectual or navigator. In the latter case the exotic nature of the union accentuates the unknown, something which is part of the dream: launching into marriage being equated with going to sea, going out into the unknown . . .

### Notes to Chapter 8

1. *Sudestasie* [South East Asia], No. 3, July 1980, p. 63.
2. R. Barthes, *Conjugales*, in *Mythologies*. Paris: Seuil (Points), 1977, p. 47.
3. Marcel Mauss, *Sociologie et Anthropologie*. Paris: PUF, 1968.
4. 'Umma' in Islam means at one and the same time people, community and nation. This concept covers all aspects, legal, political and religious.
5. In the sense attributed to it by E. Goffman: a type of attribute which brings considerable discredit on its possessor.
6. *Ethnopsychanalyse Complémentariste* [Complementarist Ethnopsycho-analysis], Paris: Flammarion, 1972, p. 134. The author makes a distinction between ethnic *personality* and ethnic *identity*.
7. *La Pensée Sauvage* [Wild Thought]. Paris: Plon, 1962, pp. 44-47.
8. In the sense in which P. Bourdieu develops this concept in his book *La Distinction* [The Distinction], Paris: Minuit edition, 1980.

# Part 3
# The Child

# 9 Becoming parents

*'We are looking for a name'*

## Expecting a Child

When I married my husband I knew and could see that he was black. I had in fact made a choice with my eyes wide open, knowing what I was letting myself in for. But the child we are now expecting is really an unknown factor (French woman, aged 24, married to a black African).

When a mixed couple are expecting a child it acts as confirmation of the choice to live together in a long-term relationship; it also marks the starting point for new questions. A third individual will bring yet another different element to this couple which is already different from others. The partners will face an endless stream of questions. The mother-to-be will be even more aware that she is in the process of 'producing' a being which is at the same time similar and yet different.

What colour will the child be? Who will he or she resemble? What about the palms of the child's hands? This added element of difference very quickly becomes an element of the unknown. The mother-to-be will certainly come into contact with young pregnant women like herself. But each of them will make her feel that 'for me it will not be the same'.

They are pregnant just like me; in that respect our experience as women is the same. But at the same time I am experiencing it all in a different way. I cannot help asking myself a thousand and one questions. I know that my child will be different to theirs. It is exciting to be distinct, but it is also unsettling.

Mixed with the unsettling feelings being experienced by this woman are the physical feelings of pregnancy. Though she may not always find the right words to describe it, she will sense an air of mystery about what is happening to her. She will see herself as a place in which an unusual person is being created. She will also wonder whether the child will be strange in some way, so different that he or she might appear unnatural. 'Don't worry, he will look like you as well', her husband responds.

Right from the beginning of pregnancy an important question will preoccupy the partners. 'What name shall we choose?' Already an attempt is being made to establish the child's identity by means of a simple vocal sound which will enable the child to be recognised as well as to recognise him or herself. Often long lists of boys' and girls' names are drawn up. In France, for instance, Jean, Marie, Pierre, Michel, Francoise, Alain, Jacques are the names which are the most frequently given to children born in Paris. The order is somewhat different in the provinces. In the Ariege region, for instance, the name Marie is used far more. But what about this child one of whose parents is from another country?

Parents show a preference for 'all-purpose' names, although the choice is never neutral. They will be careful to avoid names that are obviously Christian. They will tend to look for international or Biblical forenames. Bernard is popular in Franco-British couples, Romeo in Franco-Italian couples. Stanislas, Boris, Igor and Wenceslas seem to be favoured in marriages where one partner is from Eastern Europe, especially with Poles who have lived in France for many years. Tarik, Karim, Nassim and Ishmael, even if they point to oriental roots, will not be such a handicap as names like Mohammed or Tahar which will automatically be avoided because of their strongly Islamic connotations. There is a greater choice for girls' names. Miriam has had a staggeringly successful linguistic career in that it is used in all languages. It is also interesting to study names which end in an *a* such as Sabrina, Emma, Marina, Natasha, Raissa, Flora and Barbara. These conjure up Central European Origins. They are all to be found in the calendar. This does not stop some parents in mixed couples from inventing original names of their own, however, or from adopting regional names (e.g. Breton) to which they attribute great significance: Mikael, Ronan, Joan . . .[1].

What is actually behind the search for a name is the identity of the unborn child which starts to become a major preoccupation of the parents, grandparents and other members of the family circle. The choice of a forename will indicate the choices of lifestyle which the family must later make, choices which will significantly affect their lives. This process will reveal areas of compromise between the partners. Each of them will to an extent want to defend his or her own identity:

My husband is black. If my child is also black will I find myself living with two foreigners? I would then feel that I was the foreigner in my own home!

As each child comes along, depending on where the couple is living at the time of birth, one of the partners will experience a loss of similarity with people of his or her own nationality, whereas for the partner who is living in a foreign country the birth of the child will mean a greater sense of similarity. The exiled partner will find part of him or herself in the child, at the expense of the other partner:

I am glad my daughter's skin is a little black. It reminds me of my own country which I left a long time ago. Whenever we go back there it will be easier for her . . . (Senegalese man, aged 27).

This father is clearly expressing a far-reaching transference, with the danger of the emotional elation which the child produces in him. The child takes the foreign parent back to his personal identity and to the identity of his group.

What can you do about it? It was her choice. We let her make her own decisions, though it was hard to let go at first. It took a long time for us to accept having a black son-in-law in the family (Father of a French woman married to an African).

Opposition and reticence on the part of the family circle will be revived at the prospect of the expected birth. It will serve to remind the group of its basic, original identity, its roots:

This child is bound to be different from its cousins. After all, it's a part of Africa she's carrying in her womb.

The partners, who thought they had been quite at liberty when they married, suddenly realise the social significance their marriage takes on when it comes to descendants. Will not the child also become a pawn between them and between the societies to which they may feel they belong? They live in a real paradox: the social environment would just ignore them as mixed and may even isolate them to an extent; at the same time a greater attachment may be required of them simply because they do not fit in with the normal standard. By its arrival in their home, this child will bring them back to some fundamental questions which will work themselves out into attitudes when it comes to making choices:

The child I am expecting is already a source of joy for me. But it is something stronger than myself: I seem to be experiencing profound feelings, perhaps more so than other pregnant women. There is the problem of aesthetics. We want it to be a beautiful child and beauty is a function of various criteria which have been instilled into us. Big fair-haired people are regarded more favourably than small fair-haired people, and they are regarded more favourably than big dark people who, in turn, are regarded more favourably than small dark people. It is not a question of defects or abnormalities. It cannot be explained. It is simply what, unconsciously, we are able to accept. This child will be a living sign of the choice I made in marrying a black African. It is different, of course, for an adopted foreign child. When a woman takes a yellow or black child out, people automatically think it must be an adopted child and do not bother to ask themselves who the father might be. Indeed it is even regarded as a credit to the adoptive parents if they have adopted a foreign child. They have done a good deed. In my case, on the other hand, with a strong possibility of giving birth to a halfcaste child, I have the impression that people will say: 'What else could you expect?' It's as though I had done something wrong in marrying a black man.

The above thoughts, expressed by one woman I spoke to, clearly show how extensive and deep-rooted are the judgments of a social environment which is unprepared to accept mixed marriages. Her reference to the difference between the adopted foreign child and the halfcaste child shows what is at stake in a marriage relationships. The child she is expecting from a foreigner means that the group she belongs to has come under attack, physically touched by this foreigner with whom the group cannot easily relate. An adopted foreign child does not pose the same threat to the identity of the group. Such a child only affects the intellectual and symbolic identity, whereas the halfcaste child is perceived as an attack on its physical identity, the identity which presents the highest visible profile for the members of the group.

The desire of a mixed couple to have children is interpreted as an attack in which the social aspects of their dual relationship are clearly seen. Indeed, this wish is a more or less conscious social decision. It can range from a deliberate policy to bring together two different cultures, to a categorical refusal to have any children. The partners may want to spare children from the somewhat difficult situation they would have to live in as halfcastes.

This time before a child is born is experienced in very different ways depending on the couple in question. One expectant father, married to a Chilean woman, expresses this period of waiting very lucidly:

It came home to me that there were going to be three of us when I saw Maria getting larger. This was something real and tangible happening in her body. It triggered something in my mind. I now await the birth with an unbelievable number of questions. There are now so many of them that I don't share them all with Maria. What matters to her is that the pregnancy goes well (Frenchman, aged 28, married to a Chilean refugee).

This man confided that he had not actually thought about all these things when he first met his wife on voluntary service. Firstly, this marriage modified his previous bachelor existence: he had well and truly fallen in love. Secondly, the fact that his partner was a Latin-American refugee made certain situations more acute:

This child will be born and live the first years of his life, at least, in France. In what sense will he be Chilean?

His wife was fully engrossed in the experience she was going through. She too was twenty-eight years old and had been in Europe for six years. She had had to escape from Chile because of the repression following the coup which brought an end to the political regime of President Allende. Right from the start of her marriage she thought it inconceivable not to have children. Moreover, she saw in this child the possibility of expressing her hope in life itself. A child of challenge to counter the forces of destruction and death . . . Thus this desire to live was projected completely onto the child the couple were expecting. At no time did she ask herself questions as to the child's mixed descent and the fact that he would have a French father and a Chilean mother:

That is not at all important. There is a great deal of movement in the world. Our child will not be alone. He will be able to travel between the two countries.

Having a child drew a veil over her recent, painful past. Her husband was also optimistic, though with some reservations. Their political convictions added force to the intensity of their love which could, at times hide certain realities. The hope of a better future dominated the reality of the present and the painful objectivity of a past which was still very fresh in the woman's mind. Does this not mean that the child becomes the foundation on which hopes and plans for the future are built, as well as being a reference point for the unity of the couple which they hope to consolidate into a lasting relationship? The dynamics of their unity overcome any possibility of disunion.

It wasn't late for us to have children. We could have waited a few years. But as you can imagine, we were curious to see what our children would be like. What's more, in my society waiting is unheard of. As far as my parents are concerned they cannot see any reason for waiting (Senegalese man, aged 27).

He married Genevieve four years ago when they met at college. This young man highlights the social nature, as well as the personal nature, of the decision about having children. For the Wolof people to whom he belongs the fact of having a child confers a higher social status on an adult because it indicates that he is thereby undertaking responsibility for the continuity of the group. It shows his people that he is serious about extending the group. It also gives the group a future. In the case of mixed marriage, however, the child is not quite what the group had in mind, because the child's difference will represent an uncertainty for the partner's group. There will always be the risk of causing the child to veer towards the other group, that of the other partner:

This is the biggest question mark as I see it. What sort of life will our child have? And where will he or she live?

This father-to-be's status as an exile from his own country highlights a number of questions which all couples expecting a child ask themselves.

The future of society is uncertain. In addition, we didn't want to have children for fear of producing one more unhappy person. The desire to have children was very strong, however. We looked for excuses for living life as a twosome. Time is also passing us by: it would have to be now or never. I cannot imagine old age without children around me. It must be very sad (French woman, aged 34).

The desire to have children formulates bit by bit around an optimistic view of life. On top of this, realism may push the couple into making an emotional investment in their family life in order to counter loneliness. This is the majority view and one which is very often encouraged and given official backing. It is countered, however, by people who are adamantly opposed to having children, a view which is especially reflected in the speech of 'liberated' women. They point out the incompatibility between the quality of a couples' relationship, the choice of a demanding career, and the responsibility for bringing up one or more children:

It is more important for me to do well in my career. Every day I have to take decisions which affect society. So I can understand very well why an ordinary working woman should want to have children. It is a way of exercising real responsibility (Woman manager, aged 27, without children).

Placing their freedom of action and free time above preoccupations of child rearing, these couples are weighing up the difference in quality of life and the things they would have to give up if they were to become responsible for children. It is of course recognised that, depending on social environment and means, some couples will be able to strike a happy balance between their personal, professional expectations, and the bringing up of their children. We should also remember that many couples do not even ask themselves these questions: 'We shall just wait and see. If you knew everything in advance, you would never do anything'. In mixed couples, however, there are many partners who wonder about the consequences of their decision to have children. This preoccupation will depend on how mixed the couple is:

> I don't want any children. I'm not sure how important the fact that we are a mixed couple is in coming to this choice. But it certainly adds to the arguments. You don't even know what the future will bring for French children born today to French couples. You can imagine what it would be like for my children, marked out as physically different and with an unusual forename . . . No, I don't have the right to saddle children with such a heritage of difference. They would experience even more difficulties. I would feel I was being selfish if I had children. I would just be pleasing myself. Then I would find myself saying: 'Now you can manage by yourself'. Any children we had would be entitled to blame us for bringing them into the world (French woman, aged 30, married to a man from Mali).

Not only is this woman expressing the disinclination of social groups to integrate a child who is not just like the others, she is also highlighting the personal fears she has. The mixed nature of the couple only serves to reveal even more clearly this disinclination, though it might just be an excuse.

## The Birth

The transition from being a couple to being a family with a child is a very important time in the relationship of the partners. The period of pregnancy was in a sense a dual period in which the couple was preparing for the future. It was also an antechamber of choices. 'I don't want to forecast anything until it happens; this is one of my principles', says a young pregnant woman. Yet very soon there will be three of them.

This is not the view of a Portuguese man who has been married for three years to a woman from the Vendée region. Since they married they have got used to there only being two of them.They were happy with their independence, their weekends, their regular holidays in Portugal, etc. He is now afraid that their child will cause them to become more firmly rooted in Vendée and to become more and more cut off from Portugal. As the birth approaches, this couple thinks of the possibility of a change. The large family of the mother-to-be is already talking of the baby. This experience of the pre-birth period cannot be communicated to the expectant grandparents in Portugal, simply because of the distance involved. But they will go to see them as soon as possible after the baby has been born. As soon as they have adjusted to their new lifestyle. They will have to wait, of course, until the baby is able to stand up to the journey.

In two months the young woman will give birth for the first time. She is surrounded by sisters, cousins and parents. Her Portuguese husband has become progressively adopted into this large, closely knit family. 'He has shown himself to be as good as any other husband in the Vendée'. Nevertheless he has noticed that his relationship with his wife has tended to become less intimate, and this worries him. She seems to want to concentrate far more on the child she is expecting. It is now that he realises what a large family she has. People they had never entertained before now come to see them. The couple is looking outward. But the Portuguese husband sometimes feels the pain, not so much of loneliness, but of the fact that his own family is far away. He imagines what things would have been like if they lived in Portugal, in his own village. His family would have been omnipresent. How would his wife have put up with this? He realises how overwhelming it might be.

They badly need to be alone again. They are aware that something significant is about to happen to them as a couple. The woman knows that he will not be present at the birth. She would have liked him to, but understands his reservations which have more to do with his own personality than with his culture. 'A lot of French husbands don't like to be there when their wives give birth', she tells herself. There are some cultures in which childbirth is strictly a 'woman's affair', and men have nothing to do with it. She appreciates his solicitous attitude about countless details, his gentleness and love: 'So you still like me, even in my present condition', she says laughing.

However, he does not understand everything that is happening. For instance, he sees the relationship between his wife and the gynaecologist as somewhat unsatisfactory. He would like to know what is going on but, because of the standard of his French, he is unable to grasp some words and technical terms which he has never heard before. Knowing that he is a foreigner, he is anxious not to be an outsider in an event which involves him directly. As the father-to-be it is of interest to him. But why does the gynaecologist so rarely speak to him? Would he treat an expectant French father in the same way? His sensitiveness has grown over these last few days. He feels he is no longer indispensable for his wife and that, if need be, the birth could take place just as well without him. He can already see granny and grandpa getting their hands on the baby ... thereby taking control of his wife. He feels that his marriage is off balance. After three years of married life this is the first time he has asked such questions.

The child arrives. It is a girl. They decide to give her the single name Maria. 'Why yes, Marie — it's a lovely, uncomplicated name', says the new grandfather. 'No, it's *Maria*', replies the baby's mother, looking at her husband. The one question that had been bothering them both was whether it would be a 'normal' baby, rather than finding out if she was going to look more like her mother or her father who is typically Mediterranean to look at.

For this couple, there were not too many worries. This is not the case, however, for the partners in a Franco-African marriage, for whom the birth will be a very anxious period. The parents will find out on their first visits which features the child has inherited from its father and which from its mother.

'It's a lovely coloured child. So beautiful! Its nose isn't too wide and it has its mother's ears' (a friend of the baby's mother).

When this woman heard these remarks about her two-day old son Nicholas, she realised that her child was different and that he was already being identified by his physical features. She got on very well with her husband. They were both students and saw eye to eye in terms of ideas and tastes. But already their child, barely seven pounds in weight, the synthesis of their union, is reflecting an image of what they are as a couple. They had not seen anything in this child which would mark him out as different. But other people, even their close friends, had been quick to notice this. Later on they recognised that Nicholas did have slightly Negroid features from his father. He was the bearer of indelible distinguishing characteristics ...

The arrival of this child would to an extent upset this couple's lives. They had got used to there only being two of them and to each other. Their life together will now have to be organised differently because things have changed for them. They are happy that they have had a child together and they will now undergo a number of changes, both in their relationship and in the everyday activities of life. This child is the means whereby they make the transition from being a couple to being a family, by becoming young parents. The woman becomes a mother, and this has its tangible, physical expression in the reality of childbirth. The husband does not see things in exactly the same way. She is now fully occupied with the baby and her maternity leave enables her to stay at home, while her partner continues his normal working life, but with the new title of father.

> It was difficult because I was a young father and yet felt that our child was part of an intimate mother–child relationship from which I was excluded (the father).

This sense of exclusion was a very marked one for this man. He had had a unique relationship with his wife. They used to have many discussions on Africa, colonialism, racism, the sale of arms to South Africa, etc. This highly political couple had reached a significant consensus of ideas in many areas. Had they not both been active militants in a third-world movement? But now all this has been pushed into the background. Their first priority is now the bringing up of their child. They have to cope with such things as baby's bottles, nights of interrupted sleep, changing nappies, lowering the volume on the radio, etc. It is a new stage in life, but one which is full of new constraints.

The African husband finds it difficult to re-establish his balance. He sometimes finds it hard to understand why his wife spends so much time with the baby. 'She just seems to make work for herself'. For him, the change is not perceived in the same way. He feels that he is being pushed out in some way. He sees a stream of visitors coming through his home, people he had never seen before:

> They just turn up and I find it hard to find anything to talk about to them. I get the impression that they are merely curious to see what this child with a black father will look like. It's really the colour of his skin that they want to see.

His wife does not see things in this way. She is re-establishing old friendships which had actually fallen off when she started going out with her black student friend. She is getting the chance to see some old friends again after a gap of several years. Some of them are also married now and have children. They swap stories and advice, much of which the husband fails to appreciate. In addition he has a strange sort of feeling which is tinged with jealousy. His own family is far away and none of them is able to come and see his child. He does not tell his wife all that he is really thinking, but he is already worried about the child's future if they stay long in France. His worries are not shared by his wife. The girl he knew a few years ago is now a mother and has changed. So has he. But have they changed together?

They both feel that they will have some readjustments to make in order to maintain the quality of their relationship as a couple. The child has become the centre of their lives. It is their firstborn. Everything is new; so they make efforts. But it would seem that the mother is the one who gains in this new situation. As a French woman, she is unconsciously re-establishing her roots, through this child, and reintegrating herself with her original group and its culture. She again sets up a network of relationships, whereas the foreign husband may find himself all alone.

> It is true that I didn't give him so much attention. I was overwhelmed by the amazing thing that had happened to me. We will now arrange things differently.

There are three of them now, the cell has grown. There is a clear sense of identification with other couples who have children. An implicit sense of solidarity and certain similarities come into being ('They've got a child like the Smiths'). In an objective sense they move closer towards being an ordinary couple. Now that they have this child, they feel less different, less mixed than they were before. In their conversation the concept of being parents is implicit. The man addresses his wife, but at the same time he is also addressing the mother of his son. She, in turn, feels a greater sense of respect from her friends and colleagues. The status of mother she has suddenly acquired now overshadows her former status as the wife of a black man.

The American woman who has become a mother in a country which is not her own undergoes a return to her original identity in her home. Her husband is surprised to find her speaking to their child in English: she starts singing old songs from the West. It even seems to him that the tone of her voice is changing. She too has had to face visits from her in-laws and accept the advice of her sisters-in-law:

> I listen to them, but I find the way children are brought up in France very restrictive. It is not at all like the realm in which Asterix the Gaul operates. We are more relaxed.

The French husband is prepared to accept the somewhat strange, wild way his wife has of being a mother. She is certainly different from his three sisters. He is already quite sure that Carla, their daughter, will be different from his nieces. But this does not cause him too much concern. He is engrossed in his work. In his professional environment the birth was regarded as a normal event. He continues with his everyday routine without asking too many questions. Moreover his wife does not feel isolated. She is with her child all day long, and she has a telephone call from the States every week. He is not faced with the same type of questions as the African partner for whom the birth of a son was an intense experience, an event which gave rise to a certain sense of nostalgia and above all the regret that he could not in any social sense mark the African nature of this child because his family was not there with him. For this African, the birth was a reminder of his family's absence at his wedding when only one of his African friends and a member of his family were present.

The birth of a first child is experienced, above all, as something new which the presence of a third individual brings to the couple. It enables the couple to become less monolithic and to become more outward looking. It is in fact a return to the community which this child makes possible. But in a mixed couple it is often only one of the communities which is physically present. This presence cannot help but point to the absence of the foreign partner's family.

Right from the start the partners will have decisions to make. We have already seen how the choice of a name for the child can require lengthy discussion. After this first name has been chosen on the basis of various criteria, there is often a second name which may be just as significant, e.g. Samir, Ichem, Eddine, Jamil, David, etc. for boys, and Caroline, Catherine, Cecile for girls. This secondary name is an expression of some of the feelings which the parents have in wanting to indicate a certain attachment of the child to one or other community when the first name might indicate a preference for neutrality, distance or marked inter-nationalism. A harder decision, however, will be whether to have the child baptised for the sake of a Christian partner or to have him circumcised for a Muslim partner.

Friends with any discretion will avoid asking about such matters. The families, on the other hand, will expect the parents of the child to act in accordance with their own traditional convictions ... It is true that as regards baptism this child will remind the parents of their social *and* religious identity, even if they have given their original religious practices a wide berth. Even where the level of religious observance is very low, a certain number of religious markers persist in some families (baptism, first communion, marriage and funeral services in church). The fact that the question of baptism has been raised, or circumcision for that matter, can be seen as an indication of the real state of the convictions of each of the parents and of the relationships they have with their families on this point, with such individuals as grandparents, uncles and aunts, and with certain friends.

The fact that he is different physically from other children is only to be expected. But if he is also to differ spiritually ... (grandmother of a halfcaste child).

Moreover in many families the religious celebration of the baptism is often followed by a greater secular celebration which the guests look back on fondly.

'The grandparents won't be very happy', the young woman says when, in agreement with her Protestant German husband, she decides not to have their son Michael baptised for the time being. They had agreed to please both families by marrying on the basis of the new mixed marriage ceremony with a Protestant minister present. But they could not bring themselves to comply when it came to the upbringing of their child since they were both so uncertain about their faith themselves. As unbelievers they did not want to impose a baptism on a child incapable of deciding for itself, a baptism which in their opinion would commit him for the future: 'He can decide for himself when he is old enough'.

In the case of many mixed marriages which involve a significant difference in religion (Christian and Muslim, for example) we find ourselves confronted with the theory of *deferred choice*: that is to say, the transfer of responsibility to a choice which the child will make for itself when older. Some couples engage in interesting experiments in this regard, with or without the agreement of their ministers. But they remain the exceptions because most of them do not perform any religious ceremony. In couples where the husband is Muslim the question of circumcision for boys is a difficult one to resolve. The Muslim is deeply committed to this and his French wife cannot always understand the socio-religious significance of the practice. In some working class couples the French wife is presented with a *fait accompli* while they are on holiday in N.W. Africa. A celebration is then organised by the husband's family and this all serves to remove the emotive content from the situation. When they go back the woman will be more likely to have a pleasant memory of this ceremony. Her French family, however, will not always be so ready to understand. They will attempt to disguise their feeling of unease about what has happened to the child:

My mother wanted to know all the details. She couldn't understand how I could allow it to happen. She was quite upset by it. She now looks at my son in a different way.

Another woman accepted the fact of her son's circumcision However, she did place conditions on her husband. The 'operation' was carried out in a clinic by a surgeon they had both chosen together. A few days later they held a small celebration for some of the husband's friends who were also students in the same town as himself. It was a simple dinner and the reasons for the circumcision tended to concentrate on the hygienic, medical aspects rather than on the religious ones. However, the father was acting in accordance with his own social group's expectations. He announced it to all his family. His partner, on the other hand, was not able to invite anyone from her family. Each group has its own deeply entrenched celebrations.

The choices which the parents make in this area will be a good indication of the plans they have for the future. On a number of occasions they will have to adapt and bring their day-to-day lives into harmony with their general outlook on life. Will it be necessary for them to adopt a very strict line when it comes to taking clear-cut decisions, or will it be the very blurred area of systematic indecision? If they persist in postponing the real significance of their actions, they will run the risk of seeing irredeemable situations gradually coming into being. Will it be easier, for instance, for a child in a mixed couple to make his or her own decisions quite independently at certain points on the basis of the choices already adopted by the parents, than to start out from no choices at all? And will these be entirely without significance for the child's future after having lived for a number of years in one country and been put through school there, for example? Some parents do not hesitate in taking risks when bringing up their children. They feel it far better to do this than to be lax, which could in the long run be harmful for the child's future.

This child was born in Tunis. We didn't hesitate for a second. We had him circumcised. Then we held a celebration to show our agreement with this tradition. In this way we saved him a whole lot of problems with his school friends. They wanted to know right away whether he was like them. This did not seem in any way a problem for me, and I was able to explain it to my parents. For the same reasons we gave him a distinctly Muslim name (French woman, aged 39, married to a Tunisian).

As a committed Christian, this woman confided that this decision, taken with her husband's full agreement, was also consistent with her wish to be integrated into this N.W. African country. As she saw it, it was necessary, at all costs, to put down strong roots based on tangible situations, and above all not to put her child in a difficult position or in situations which were difficult to interpret because plans had been made in such a vague manner. As far as she and her husband were concerned, choices had to be made now and not in the future. Other parents are less definite and prefer to leave the child a margin of freedom: 'At least he won't be able to blame us later on'. They think that choices must be made by the child when it becomes capable of doing so. 'He can choose for himself when he is older'. In both types of choice advantages and disadvantages will be encountered. There could never be a theory which applied to all mixed children irrespective of their individual personalities, characters, sex, position in the family and personal tastes, and taking into account how the parents see the child's future unfolding.

**Notes to Chapter 9**

1.  I have come across the same form of name giving in parents adopting children of foreign origin. The slow process of choosing the forename(s) tells us a lot about how important what they stand for actually is for the individual bearing that name, for his or her family and for the whole social group.

# 10 Education and difficult choices

*'When he's bigger, he can choose for himself'*

The lives of mixed couples are continually beset with what are sometimes difficult decisions. These often mark the limits of sharing between the partners who will at such times express views from their own privileged positions. They may also unconsciously compete with one another. One of them will take decisions alone when the other does not have the time to enter into discussion. Difficulties can arise when the couple has one or more children. Already at the waiting stage, when the woman is pregnant, certain questions will be raised. Later when the child goes to school and takes exams, the parents will have to face up to even more complex situations, until the point at which the child is able to make his or her own choices. What religion and what nationality will the children adopt?

The choices made earlier by the parents will channel the directions opted for by the young people. In the same way, if they have refrained from influencing such choices, they may have created situations of empty choices or situations in which decisions are absent. One tends to take account of one's heritage when choosing one's way through life. Indeed, earlier choices made by the parents in place of the child, when the child was too young to make a decision, may avoid the stressful position of being faced with a labyrinth of situations which would be even more difficult to unravel. Might it not be more difficult to change options than to be able to make decisions with a certain amount of serenity? Instead of the void created by the absence of choice, a background of not altogether finalised decisions can lead a child to a well considered conclusion, to the point of maturity. It is certainly a difficult task to maintain one's sense of balance as one lives through this progression of choices. It cannot be denied that there is a marked interdependence between the choices made by the adult parents and those of the child as he or she grows up.

The child grows up in a family, sometimes with brothers and sisters. He is aware of himself, of his position in the family group. He also lives in other environments, particularly that of school. He will come up against situations in which his friends may tell him that he is different.

To begin with we were the only Americans in the school. Then we were treated like stars; when they saw us coming, 200 yards away, they would shout 'Here come the Americans'. I soon got used to it and made a number of friends (Patrick, aged 11, American father, French mother).

This child was aware of the fact of being different. He was even proud of it. Another child, in contrast, will blame its parents for having married one another:

'But why did you marry an Arab, mummy?'

This is the title of an article which appeared in a Moroccan daily.[1] It was the subject of a sometimes heated exchange of letters over a number of days in that same journal. This title was only picking up on the views expressed in a 1979 Radio France programme by a Moroccan father, originally from Casablanca, but living in France.[2] He was speaking about his mixed marriage with a certain amount of sadness, if not bitterness. He was now on the point of getting divorced and explained the reasons why he and his wife had come to this decision.

Following an argument between my wife and myself, I was deeply hurt when my six year old son asked his mother 'Why did you marry an Arab, mummy?'

He will hear the reactions of those around him. In what ways will he be different from the others? Will he be closer to foreign children? Or to French children if he lives in France? He will internalise a number of images projected onto him by his friends and teachers, and his identity will take shape as a result of a labyrinth of circumstances for which the parents are responsible. He will identify with them in the situations they actually live through. Although they would like the child to be aware of belonging to two groups, possibly with dual nationality, will it not be the case that school, daily experience and institutions will align the child with whatever is the dominant norm?

Might it not be possible that the child becomes treated like a pawn in a game if the parents are not careful to check their own selfish wishes? Whether consciously or unconsciously, they could influence and push the child one way or the other. The child may also be treated as a pawn between the societies when the balance of cultural and economic forces is a very critical one. There may sometimes be historic relationships between the groups which perpetuate the situation in which one is dominant and the other dominated.


## The Surname

The giving of a name at the time of birth had set in motion a spirit of conciliation between the partners. But it also gave rise to a number of questions, particularly between the mixed couple and their respective families.

The time will come when the child becomes aware not only of forenames but also of his or her surname. It is usual in many countries that the father's (foreign) name is used. The realisation will come of being the biological child of the father and that a foreign surname is a symbol of someone who is different from other fathers. The child will ask the mother what her name was before she was married. She may give the impression of a woman who is happy with the name of the child's father:

> Our name sounds a bit Italian. People often ask me its origin and discover that I'm married to a Moroccan.

One mother had noticed on a number of occasions a certain disguised racism when people learned that she was married to a N.W. African, so she had done all she could not to announce the fact to anyone she met. She had also adopted the habit of hiding or camouflaging the fact. She would write her name with a *y* at the end instead of an *i*. She would often add her own (very French) surname to her married name. 'Why do they call you that, mummy?' her daughter asked. 'Because it's my real name'. So the other name, that of the child's father is a false name? This woman had not realised that she was introducing an element of doubt into her daughter's emerging sense of identity. She acted, albeit unconsciously, as though she were in fact denying the existence of the father because he was a foreigner. In this way she reveals her desire that her child should not be seen as foreign, because of the social difficulties it involves and because of the somewhat intolerant majority group. But the child needs to know the whole truth and her father must speak to her in order that the mother — who represents the majority group — should not have the dominant influence. This difficult balance needs to be maintained at the precise moment when the child is developing his or her identity. This requires a certain amount of self-denial on the part of both of the parents.

One child began to understand that his surname and forename had certain 'effects' on people. His teachers were discreet about it, but this was not always the case when it came to the public authorities and when he went to high school. The people who worked with him even thought that his 'unusual' forename confirmed his physical type which was different from other children. They would often add: 'It's not surprising that he's unstable and undisciplined'.

This perception of a person's surname and forename may be expressed in ambiguous ways. It depends to a great extent on the welcome a person receives from those he or she comes into contact with and also on the way that person's parents relate to their name. Is it unique in the area where they live or is it fairly common? It may be a surprise when people hear it for the first time.

Once people have heard my name for the first time, there's no longer any problem. It's like a sort of barrier I have to get across. People need to know and then make their own judgment. It's never the same after (Tarik, aged 17, Moroccan father).

The reactions of girls in this respect are different. They know that if they marry, they will lose their surname. The fact of having, say, an Arab surname may give rise to unpleasant thoughts, and often to an expression of curiosity:

I made a great effort to understand; then I simply became Nadia, especially with my friends. At the same time, I wondered whether they knew what my surname was, that is to say my father's name. But I suppose that this even happens to French children (Nadia, aged 18, Moroccan father).

Nadia also related that there is an important reason for this: her parents do not come into contact with her friends'' parents. There is therefore no reason or need to retain her surname, apart from the fact that it is a difficult one to hold on to. 'What's more, one day I will lose it. Few people will actually have known what my name was. Everyone knows me as Nadia', she added. This is not the case for her brothers who will keep their surname unless they change or modify it. All their lives they will have to cope with what will at times be hostile reactions, and inspections of their identity cards which will sometimes make them appear as foreigners. They also know that they will pass on this inherited name to their own children, whereas the daughters will have an opportunity of getting rid of their embarrassing surname.

In a mixed marriage, a woman who refuses to take on her husband's surname introduces what can sometimes be a serious doubt in her child's mind. By rejecting it, she is in a sense devaluing it, because in some countries she is legally entitled to use her own surname. The child will find it difficult to assess properly the situation as a result of the father's name being in some sense denied, for children have a great need for structural unity. This ambiguity, which may only be an insignificant matter, will take on exaggerated proportions for the children who will make judgments on the basis of their immature subjectivity and sensitivity to the moment. Will they too have double surnames? Their friends will latch onto this double surname and ask various questions:

> I could sense their curiosity and was aware that I was unusual, that my parents were not like everyone else's (French girl, aged 15, daughter of a Franco–N.W. African mixed marriage).

This girl described to me her experiences in forming relationships. Whenever she met someone for the first time she had to give an explanation of her background. This was the case with friends, with teachers and even later on in life. Especially when she started going out with boys. She was even aware that there was a 'before' and 'after' to relationships.

> I went out with a pleasant boy. I liked him a lot. We met at a school party. He was from a different school. We just knew one another by our first names. My name, Andrée, didn't cause any suspicion. We saw each other again over the next two days and became very close. We already knew a lot about each other. We even began to flirt. We only thought about ourselves and our friends. We never spoke about our parents. But then he said: 'I don't even know what your surname is'. I told him. 'What?' he said, 'You mean you're Algerian?' 'No, I'm French', I said, 'my father's Algerian'. I immediately noticed a change in him. It had a deep effect on me.

She felt very strongly about the fact that her surname was not a neutral one. Her father's surname caused reactions in people. This was a big lesson for her to learn. She now tells people her full name from the outset. In this way she is able to form real friends from the start. She does not engage in any form of deception. Everyone knows who her father is.

This story illustrates very well the social value of a surname. If the forename is an indication of the private personality, the father's surname places an individual in a social, generic (not to say genetic) grouping, in a whole history of experience and in a heritage. The forename is an individual element grafted onto the overall identity. Although she was thought highly of, accepted, liked and courted for herself, Nadia was kept at a distance because of her N.W. African name. Her personality was doubled and even denied by the whole system of value judgments which her surname produced in the range of positive and negative feelings displayed in people's reactions to foreigners of various nationalities. It is quite certain that if this young woman had had an Anglo-Saxon sounding surname her partner would not have reacted in the same way, unless he already had some reason for not liking Anglo-Saxons. He would of course have been curious about her background, but it is doubtful whether this would have caused him to change his whole attitude to her. The father's name, in many societies at least, becomes the family name which is passed on from generation to generation. It is used as a reference point for affiliation and each member of the family is identified on the basis of this surname (administratively and legally, etc.). This system is, of course, unfair on women, the mothers of families, when it operates on an exclusive basis, as is the case in some countries. But this is not always merely a question of the name one bears; it can also be understood in terms of the sharing of responsibility by husband and wife.

The name will be one element among others which will enable the child to find his or her place in society. It will, however, be the major tangible element in early childhood for the establishing of an identity and personality. Gradually the child will move from the stage of more or less voluntary, unconscious acceptance of a given name to the more conscious stage of choosing a name for oneself and having other people use that name. The path towards autonomy has begun . . .

Son or daughter of X and Y . . . The forename and surname have already given an indication of a dual affiliation. Other questions will arise, particularly with regard to education, and these will be areas in which the children will have to establish an identity in areas in relationship to themselves, their parents and their friends. The answers to these questions will involve the expression of solidarity, to a greater or lesser degree, with the groups to which the parents belong. Children are actually a social link that no-one had imagined. They reawaken the identity of the parents: religious, cultural, national. They remind each partner of the group to which they belong. But what about the children themselves? To which group will they become attached? This is an important issue between the partners: the children are tangible proof of the sharing of power within the couple. They will be affected by the two parents and by their families, and will allow themselves to be influenced by them to a certain extent.

In many mixed couples the parents might tend to adopt attitudes of withdrawal or abdication when it comes to questions about their children's future. They may even evade the issue by transferring the choices to be made, i.e. escape by transferring the whole burden of deferred choice onto the children. The children will then be left to act consciously for themselves when they are able to act independently. But the parents often fail to realise that choices are made on the basis of experiences the children have had in the family and outside of the home, be it in terms of language, when they go to school in a given country; religion, when they are more or less integrated into religious practices along with friends of their own age; or in terms of nationality, when they have been living in one country for a number of years. The place in which the parents choose to live will be a decisive factor.

Does this mean that the education of a child from a mixed marriage is specific? And if so, in what sense? It is impossible to give a categorical answer to this fundamental question. There are as many different situations as there are different social conditions in which mixed couples live.

Education is indeed an important issue in the sharing of power and adjustments couples have to make. It will be closely linked with where the family lives and with the different ages of the children. Will the family live in the father's country or the mother's country? Will it be in the U.S.A., Hungary, Tunisia, Sicily, Germany or Great Britain that the child is to spend his or her early years? This will depend much on the relationship between the partners as well as on the relationship between the individual partner and the society in which he or she lives. What status does the parent have as a man or woman? What were relationships between the two countries like in the past? Were they cordial or hostile? Have there been any wars resulting in confrontation between the countries for a number of years, as in the case of France and Germany, France and Algeria, or the U.S.A. and Vietnam? In what way does a history of poor relations between a dominant country and the dominated country over several decades of colonialism affect the lives of a mixed couple and the lives of their children?

Moreover, the importance and nature of the educational infrastructure in the country of residence will have varied consequences. Depending on the social environment these will have a more or less decisive effect on the learning of language, on the direction the children's education is to take, and on secondary or higher education. Will it not be difficult for the children if, for one reason or another, the parents change their location? Living in France, the children will have more opportunities to learn English, but less opportunity to learn Arabic if they live in a small provincial town. They may become disoriented if they are suddenly taken to live in N.W. Africa because their father is obliged to return to his own country for professional reasons. The children will be confronted with a sort of alternating bilingualism, unless the couple settle down for good in one country. Is it possible to be sure that such a choice is final?

Thus the education of the children will be conditioned by family, school and location factors. These three elements are closely linked. Indeed, depending on the place of residence the social/family environment may be completely different: what is a reduced, nuclear family in France may become an enlarged family elsewhere. This is often the case, for instance, for Franco-Islamic couples. When they return to an Islamic country, the children discover an enlarged family group: grandparents, uncles, aunts, cousins. The context will be different again if the father happens to be a Californian. . .

Might it be the case that what distinguishes the child from a mixed marriage from another child of the same social environment, is the fact that he or she is not always sure of living in the same place, because one of the parents is foreign? Moreover, when it comes to the education of this child, do the partners in a mixed marriage give equal chances to the complementary cultural and ethnic aspects of their relationship? Is it not likely to be the case that an Algerian worker will allow himself to be dominated by his French wife who is from a marginally higher social class than his own? Will he sometimes react with an uncontrolled authoritarianism or with resignation? What sort of educational autonomy will this couple come up with? What will make up the French, N.W. African, or American element in that education, at what time, for which child and in what location? What identification system will the child refer to?

The choice of a forename was already indicative of a certain complexity and involved a certain amount of dialogue between the partners as to the identity of the child. Added to this, as we have seen, is the surname which can also at times be the subject of questions in the mind of the child. When it comes to education, the parents' choices, even if they seem tame ones, will never be neutral. These choices are consolidated on the basis of the sex of the child, as well as on the basis of the more or less conscious intentions of the couple to settle or re-settle in one or other country. Will the child find him or herself between the two cultures, as though sitting on a trapeze? Will the child opt for one in preference to the other? Or will the child live equally in two cultures, in the same way as one can enjoy two landscape views at once when travelling in a railway compartment? Will he or she then live in a third country? What will the child's roots be? There are many questions to be answered and there are not always ideal solutions to them.

The children of mixed marriages pose a difficult question on two levels: between the parents and between the societies to which their parents belong. They are in effect an objective link between the educational colourings of each of the parents and of the social environments.

Education is the action carried out by the adult generations on those not yet mature enough for social life. The purpose is to instil into the child a number of physical, intellectual and moral states which are required of him both by the political society as a whole and by the particular environment for which he is destined.[3]

Émile Durkheim defined education in these terms in a text written in 1922, highlighting the overall aspects of education and not just the parental expectations. Can we speak of a 'mixed state' of education for such a child, or are the differentiating influences of social environment more significant? What common experience is there between the child of a N.W. African father who is a skilled worker in a metal company, and the child of another N.W. African who happens to be an embassy adviser? The latter will have more in common with upper class children, whereas the former will be closer to the working classes with whom he or she lives in close contact. Nevertheless against this educational background there are also specific cultural elements from which the child will be able to benefit all the more if he or she is from a higher social class. The leisure activities of these two children will have nothing in common. When on holiday in N.W. Africa they will experience two quite different social realities. Comparison is even more difficult when the children are of different nationalities.

Last summer we went to America for a month. I was very glad because I met my old friends again and didn't want to come back. I would like to go back to America next year. In February I'm going skiing for a week and it'll be fun. The other summer we went to Germany for two weeks, to Holland, Belgium and Britain. I've been to thirteen different countries ... This summer we're going to Scotland and England (Patrick, aged 11, American father).

This boy is clearly expressing a point of view about a privileged environment. The 'mixed state' here is a highly valued one. This would not be the case for a boy from a modest family who would only rarely have an opportunity to visit the foreign country in which his grandparents live. Thus it can be seen that the parents are not always in control of the education of their children, even if they cherish certain privileges.

Children will not in reality live between two worlds, between two countries and between two cultures. They will actually live in one country or the other for certain periods of their lives, within an intimate family context, and will be governed by various social bodies which will have a considerable *formative influence* on them, of which they will be the products.[4] They will be more or less socially integrated in a society or social group at a given point in time. If this setting changes, for whatever reason, they will need to work hard over a certain period of time in order to adapt. But this adaptation does not so much have to do with such specific areas as the difference of culture, language, religion or nationality. The experience of belonging to a group is also defined by everyday practices and customs which children have in common with their classmates and friends, as well as by activities engaged in at informal or organised clubs and associations. The children have to integrate a whole series of values 'in an unavoidable situation which is backed up by the whole force of society'.[5] They are therefore also caught between two societies. They will actually inherit the social positions assumed by their parents in their marriage relationship, which in turn is linked up with the societies from which they come. Both parents will transmit standards to their children, of both a social and a general nature, and these will be relayed or taken over by school and various social groups.

Will the children therefore belong more to one country than to the other? How will the children feel about this? And what about the parents?

## Religion

What will the child's religion be? Whether he or she lives in France or Germany, the child from a mixed couple, in which the French mother is Catholic and the German father Protestant, will not find it very difficult to find space between these two confessions, because they are very close to one another. However real obstacles can arise in some very traditional areas where the level of religious practice is high. Nevertheless the Christian churches have been engaged in open ecumenical dialogue for the last few decades and this has smoothed over a number of areas of conflict. This does not of course make it any easier for a child to be able to say Protestant *and* Catholic when it comes to purely legal matters.

In the case of a Franco–N.W. African couple living in Africa, the influence of the larger family will be less intense in a city like Algiers or Casablanca than in a rural region of Southern Tunisia. The child will be taken firmly in hand right from birth. As we have already seen, the choice of the forename will already have marked the child with a religious identity. The French mother will be helpless to oppose the circumcision of her son without risking a breakdown in the relationship with her husband's family. This N.W. African ritual is considered normal practice and is tied up with social promotion and integration of the child with those of his own age group. It is quite common in certain schools for the child to be examined by his classmates, when they are having a P.E. lesson for instance. One mother related how her son thought this was a form of bullying. She was not overstating the case. Previously his friends had sometimes called him the 'son of the French woman', in a jeering fashion. But as soon as they realised that 'he was like them', he became one of them and there was no longer any problem.

It is better for such children to be circumcised if they are to live in N.W. Africa. Even if the father is prepared for the child to be brought up as a Christian, circumcision is really unavoidable (Mother).

This woman, a practising Catholic, had lived for fifteen years in a Tunisian city. She and her Tunisian husband had a balanced relationship. She had chosen many years back that they should settle in this country. She went through the various choices that both she and her husband, as well as the children, had to make; and she did so with a serenity which was based on her initial decision.

The very varied situations in which mixed couples live make it impossible to lay down any guidelines in the area of religion. The social context of daily life during a lengthy stay in a country must be taken into account when family decisions have to be taken. One Franco-American couple were living in France when they decided to have their children baptised into the Catholic religion. When they returned to the U.S.A., the children went to a Baptist church in the suburbs of Washington, the place where they were then to live. Another Franco-Madagascan couple chose to have their children baptised rather than leave them the choice of doing so for themselves when they were older.

There are in fact two types of situation. Either the environment in which the family lives is very permissive and is not bothered by the fact that the children have not been baptised; or else it is intolerant and restrictive, urging the parents to conform with the commonly accepted rules. In the first case there is comparative freedom. In the second case social constraint takes precedence. The parents' hesitation is under-standable, of course, but it can also have serious consequences for the child later on. Would it not be better to have a child quickly circumcised when he is very young (by a surgeon in a clinic) than to saddle him with serious problems in terms of affiliation, identity and integration into a group later on, if there is the likelihood of his living in N.W. Africa?

A young black woman and a French student, both of them atheists, are actively engaged in an extreme left movement. They do not see why they should impose a religious mark on their child since they flatly reject any religious ideology. They resist the pressures from their respective families with whom they have little to do. But they also recognise the fact that their child has grandparents ... When the child is old enough for catechism, he may want to join with his friends in the same parish, especially if one of his parents practices his or her religion.

> Every Sunday I saw my mother go to mass. I sometimes went with her of my own free will. It was my choice. And I must admit I was attracted by what I heard. We would also talk about it at meal times with my father. He had nothing against it; his own religious practice as a Muslim was limited to the bare essentials (Nadia).

One priest I interviewed on the matter of catechism for children of mixed parents in Islamic countries gave me his own point of view. There would seem to be no official doctrine. Each family comes up with its own context for religious faith based on the situations they actually ex-perience: 'Everyone is involved in the search: the bishops, the priests, committed religious people, the parents and ... even the children'. The success of a couple's relationship is one factor in favour of religious harmonisation. The children's happiness or sense of well-being is linked up with their becoming rooted in the country. Later on they will be responsible adults who must create a synthesis of Arab/Muslim values and the values of the gospels. The latter would tend more towards bringing about a lifestyle of Christian authenticity without a triumphal label.

This priest was not therefore in favour of producing children kept apart from the others and receiving a syncretic religious education: this would amount to nothing more than a compromise which would water down the specifics of each religion. He was more in favour of a double exposure and integration into the two religions which would highlight the possible areas of agreement and the areas of irredeemable disagreement as the different theologies stand. Why should they not be 'the inventors of a new way of living out a faith in Jesus' in a specifically Muslim context ... ?

This point of view from the other side of the Mediterranean echoes the search being engaged in here in Europe among Muslim–Christian couples. Some parents present their children with a special catechism which emphasises the close relationship of religions, based more on the Old Testament than on the New. There is a frequent reference to Abraham, whereas less emphasis is given to the specifics of Christian doctrine such as the Trinity or the divine nature of Jesus Christ. In several places a search for bridges between the two religions has been encouraged by the SRI (Secretariat for Relations with Islam) which has been in operation for a number of years following Vatican II.[6] The religious experience of this Franco-N.W. African child will therefore be a complex one. It is often the slightest practice on the part of the parents which, at least for a number of years, masks adherence to a religious identity.

'All his cousins have made their profession of faith, but Jabril hasn't', my mother said to me one day on the telephone. She had suddenly realised that he wasn't like her other grandchildren (A mother).

Some situations are very rich in experiences when the families recognise that the children do not belong to them as though they were personal property, but that they must independently go their own way in life through a series of moral and religious choices.

## Language

The choice of language is less involved, but it does have practical consequences. It depends basically on the context in which the couple lives. The language spoken in everyday life is not a neutral practice. Words, in their apparent ordinariness, indicate a way of thought. And the language learned by children in a mixed family will structure their way of thinking and the way in which they act.

When we came to France we were only going to stay for nine months. They only spoke English at home although they understood French. Their grandmother told them to speak French to me and to their father so that they would get used to it before their return to the United States. It wasn't easy and they didn't manage too well. Then she offered to give them twenty centimes for every day in which they spoke French at home. After that they always spoke French at home. This year, by contrast, it is a question of getting them to speak English at home so that they won't forget their mother tongue. So at Christmas I proposed a change-over: in light of inflation it was to be five Francs a week if they spoke English. It is working: they are speaking English, especially Patrick who always needs money . . .

As presented here in the words of this mother of two Franco-American children, the problem does not seem so dramatic. Arrangements are made here for enabling the children to find a happy medium between their two languages. Humour and a judicious system of motivation are not ruled out . . . It is quite clear that French was becoming the dominant language in that it was spoken at school, with friends and in daily conversations with shopkeepers. This only leaves the family to balance out the situation by using the other language.

In the case of a mixed Franco-N.W. African couple, however, is there not the risk of placing one language at an advantage, i.e. Arabic in N.W. Africa and French in France? On the other hand a child in a mixed marriage in which the father is a top manager in a N.W. African country, will have more opportunities of speaking French with the parents: the father is bound to speak French, so the child will speak French as a first language, since this is the language in which the couple communicate. A basic knowledge of Arabic will be communicated by members of the family (grandparents) until the day when this language is learnt at school or college. This assimilation of the Arabic language will be speeded up if the child lives in a rural environment, especially if the father is from this type of background.

There may therefore be widely differing situations, depending on the couples themselves and on the places where they live. Nevertheless, the linguistic element will always be an important one, because the children will belong to the culture of the language which they speak most fluently. For language is not just a social code for communication; it is a whole mixture of feelings, thoughts and ideas which are significant to the speaker. They are 'affected by the words'[7] they utter in the sense that, through those words they establish relationships with things, events and situations.

I often tell my son to go and fetch water from the fountain (N.W. African father).

The fact of saying *fountain* instead of *tap* is linked up with a linguistic context which is anchored in a social and geographic environment which is in turn linked up with a childhood in which he would often see his sisters going to the village fountain for water in Kabylia where he was born.

I've corrected him on this for fifteen years now, and it has no effect. He still says fountain. It just makes us laugh now (his wife).

The marking of time is also different, depending on whether one is using, say, French or Arabic. Past, present and future in French do not find exact equivalents in the Arabic completed and uncompleted tenses. Where in French an event has happened, is happening here and now, or will happen, in Arabic this event will either be regarded as completed or uncompleted. The French-speaking father will have a cultural affinity with the French, but does it reach as far as his emotions and thought patterns? Many examples from the German language show that there are differences, particularly with respect to masculine and feminine genders.

Is it the case that the child of a bilingual couple will have two mother tongues? This is a difficult question, all the more so because linguists are discovering various sorts of bilingualism in children whose parents have the same language. For the children of a mixed marriage the status of each partner's language also depends on the communication situation within a given geographic context. However, if one refers to the most orthodox psychoanalytical theory, it is important that the father's language is not too devalued in the child's system of symbolic representation. The parents' awareness of this will play an important role, especially in connection with the search for compensatory factors and for a balance within the marriage relationship and in the status of each parent as the child sees it. In the case of a Franco-N.W. African (or Franco-African) couple who are living abroad in the husband's country, the French mother will have times of intimate conversation with her children and will more often than not speak French to them. It is later on at school, though already in contact with playmates, that the child will gain full access to a different linguistic orientation. He or she will then acquire the words, expressions and sometimes even the whole grammatical system and vocabulary with which to express themself in both languages.

If the bilingualism is balanced, the child may acquire the ability of adapting to another world, understanding the way in which the other person thinks, especially at home. The other person, in this case, is the father with whom the child will experience a greater sense of closeness than before. It is then perhaps that the French wife will feel the need to learn Arabic herself, if she had not done so before. Indeed, if she fails to do so, it may be difficult for her to accept being excluded linguistically from this parent–child dialogue. In cases where the French-speaking child becomes Arabic speaking, does this mean that their personality changes as a result of having access to two different thought patterns? It would be necessary to carry out a careful analysis of his or her linguistic habits. Which language is normally spoken? On what subjects and with whom? It would also be necessary to consider how lessons and leisure time (cinema, television, radio, records) are divided up between Arabic and French. What linguistic use does he or she make of their time? And with whom do they spend this time?

I tend to keep to my French friends. They don't speak Arabic of course. This has always been the case ... (Nadia).

This high school girl, who attends a French lycée, is closer to her French classmates and friends than to her Arab acquaintances. She is studying Arabic, however, and speaks it with her father. The example of the American children in France is the same. Their classmates are all French. Only at home do they speak any English. This was such a cause of concern for their parents, as we saw above, that they looked for ways, including financial inducements, of encouraging them to speak English.

Does the fact of switching over from one language to another, that is to say having varying language habits, produce any special sensitivity in the child?

I speak both languages; perhaps I speak French better. However I feel more at ease in Arabic in certain circumstances: when I'm talking about Islam with my friends or when talking about the sort of cooking I like. At those times I naturally want to use Arabic words. I am better able to express what I really feel. On the other hand, when I think of an aeroplane, I tend to say it in French, or I simply say the word 'Boeing'. As you can see, certain things influence the way I think (highschool boy, aged 16, French mother).

The description given by this boy, the child of a mixed marriage, points out certain limits to his bilingualism. If he speaks about cooking in Arabic it is perhaps because, living in N.W. Africa, he has been strongly influenced by the everyday food he is used to eating in an enlarged family atmosphere, which has given rise to this linguistic preference. But it is in French (or should we say 'Franglais') that he speaks about an aeroplane. Might this be the recollection of past experience, e.g. a holiday in France when he travelled in a Boeing aircraft? It is quite understandable that Arabic words are conceptually suited to a discussion of Islam by which he may be profoundly influenced, as though he had never left N.W. Africa.

'They can't eat anything without putting ketchup on it' (French mother, American father).

A family of Franco-American children surprise their French friends whom they have invited to lunch. They seem to put ketchup on all their food. They even eat it on bread as though it were jam. I myself was surprised when I first saw Americans in the restaurant at the Smithsonian Institute, Washington, queuing with a plate of chips in their hands so that they could douse it with ketchup from a tap specially designed to dispense this condiment. It is quite clear that the word ketchup does not have the same connotations for a Frenchman as it does for an American. Depending on one's culture, one will react to words in a different way. In the setting of a mixed home, however, a child will experience different communication situations, whereas outside of the home he or she will be more or less obliged to conform to the use of the dominant language of the country.

My father was English, half Irish actually: my mother is French. The first language I learned was English until the age of eight; then came French. My early years, from the age of two to eight, were spent in England. So that was the first language I assimilated and absorbed without conscious effort. I realised this affinity with English when I first had to play in English: I was able to do it with ease and with unbelievable pleasure, as though this language were in my soul, able to come out effortlessly; French, on the other hand, always gives me problems; I don't express myself very well in French; it is not a clear language; it seems to have a poor composition and a poor orthographic system: I'm always making errors in construction due to the fact that I'm translating from English. It's very complicated (extract from an interview with Michael Lonsdale[8]).

Having been deeply influenced by his early childhood spent in England, Michael Lonsdale, the French actor, clearly states his views on the differences between the two languages he uses. He is much more at ease when using the English language. It is not surprising that this actor should be well known for his interpretations of radio texts. As Lonsdale himself says, 'it's the intensity with which you say "it's beautiful" that expresses your emotion. In France you would have to use additional words before and after. The French say: "Oh . . . que c'est beau" ( . . .), or: "Ah, que je suis content de vous voir . . .". The Englishman will say: "I'm *so* happy to see you . . .". Lonsdale clearly shows a certain division between different areas of language, a separation between a vehicular, somewhat functional, language, and a language for emotional communication.

However, it is often also the case that speech is mixed according to the subject under discussion: words and expressions from one or other language trigger off a chain of words. This qualified use of bilingualism is experienced differently depending on the social environments to which one belongs and on the languages used. Some languages are thought highly of, e.g. English or German, particularly in the upper classes where the learning of such languages is encouraged by means of frequent trips or periods spent in the countries where those languages are spoken. Moreover, sending their children to 'good schools' will be one policy adopted by those who can afford it in order to enhance such a bilingual education, whereas in other social classes the children will go to an ordinary school like everyone else, be it in France, the U.S.A., Germany or N.W. Africa.

There will therefore be a great difference between the child of an immigrant father, going to a primary school in the Paris region where more than 50% of pupils are of foreign origin, and the child of a professional Tunisian father in the centre of Tunis, going to the Mutuelville lycée which provides education for French and foreign children whose parents are government officials, teachers, managers, embassy attachés, etc.

Religion and language are two determining factors in the education of children from mixed marriages. There may be great differences between two individuals who have been brought up in two different systems. These are accentuated by the social position of the parents, or the social position of either partner in the social hierarchy of the country in which they live. But there are other questions facing these children within the family framework itself. Particularly when there are a number of children of different sexes, divisions will tend to be made quite naturally with respect to each partner and each member of the family. One child may be more American or more Asian, and another child may be more French, depending on whether the child is a boy or a girl, an older or younger child, and depending on whether they were born in Newport, Saigon or Vichy. Each child will be subject to the influence of a given lifestyle on the basis of his or her position in the family. The place in which the family happens to live will also be a decisive factor in determining certain tastes and aptitudes which a child will acquire at a time in his or her life when very receptive to the influences of a close family setting, as well as those of other significant environments (friends, school, games, sports, etc.). The child is plunged alternately into several 'cultural baths' and each of them colours him or her to a certain extent.

## Nationality

If the choice of nationality can be made when the child is older, there will remain one more important question to be answered by the parents, and by the child himself.

'They have dual nationality'.
'I told them they had dual nationality'.

For a number of years the children from a mixed marriage enjoy the status of dual nationality. However, the two nationalities cannot be exercised simultaneously. Thus the son of a Franco-American couple will be French while they are living in France, his mother's country. If he returned to the U.S.A., he would then be American. A child whose parents are both American, on the other hand, will remain American even if they live in France.

'As far as nationality goes, Nadia will make her own choice if she is allowed to'.

When the child reaches the age of majority, he or she will be asked to make a choice. This may pose various problems, particularly if the decision involves the obligation to perform military service in either of the countries concerned. The duration can vary: it may be a single or a double term, and it commits an individual to a national community. The boy born in to a Franco-N.W. African family will often find it hard to understand the need to go off to the southern Saharan region for a number of months in order to engage in military training manoeuvres which all Algerians of his age have to undergo.

If the mother, of French origin, has become a naturalised citizen in a N.W. African country, she may thereby have demonstrated a commitment to her husband's country, or she may simply have expressed her commitment without giving up her French nationality and cultural origins. As far as their children are concerned, they will be regarded as citizens of the N.W. African partner's country. In they eyes of the law they will not be allowed to leave that country without their father's permission. They may even become pawns in difficult situations, particularly if the husband and wife are going through a stormy phase in their relationship. The problem may become insoluble and force the mother to stay in her husband's country so that she can be close to her children until they reach the age of legal majority.

To a certain extent the fact of having dual nationality increases one's problems. From a purely legal point of view, the child of a French mother has French nationality; this is definitely the case if the child is born in France. If the child is born abroad, he or she may give up this nationality by making a declaration to that effect before a magistrate or a French consul abroad. French nationality will actually be retained unless he or she decides to give it up on obtaining majority. All countries confer their nationality on a child born to a father from that country. Children with a French mother and a Spanish father, even if they are born in France, will also have Spanish nationality. In the same way, they might also be Portuguese, Italian, Algerian, Moroccan, etc. They actually have two nationalities and each country considers them to have its own nationality. They will therefore be French in France and Italian in Italy, i.e. subject to both French law *and* Italian law. Common legislation is slowly taking shape with some countries: Belgium, the United Kingdom, Spain, Italy, Luxembourg, Israel and Switzerland.

Nationality has other effects, however. Children will normally take their father's surname. In Spain, on the other hand, these children will have a double surname, the father's following that of the mother. In West Germany the partners can choose a common surname for their children. Moreover, if each partner retains his or her original nationality, the children's surnames will be determined by the place in which the family lives. They will usually have the father's surname. In addition to this, parental authority is recognised jointly in families where the partners are of the same nationality. If they are of different nationalities, however, the law of the place where they reside will be applicable in the event of any dispute between them. Thus Tunisian or Algerian law will be the sole arbiter in determining the rights of each partner if the couple lives in Tunisia or Algeria. If each lives in his or her own country, the judge will apply the law of the country in which the matter was taken to court. Moreover, the respective rights of husband and wife are different from one country to another. The Hague Convention of 5 October 1961 laid down the jurisdiction of legal authorities with particular reference to the protection of minors. But not all countries subscribe to this convention . . .

## Place of Residence

Before reaching the age of majority, the child will be wholly subject to the considered (or sometimes conflicting) wishes of the parents. As we saw earlier, the place of residence is a decisive factor in the child's life. It is important in how choices are made: religion, language, nationality, education, etc. If the parents do not have a fixed residence, the children will have to get used to changes until able to choose where to live for themselves.

'At the moment we speak French, but I want him to learn Arabic, both spoken and written' (Moroccan woman, aged 25, married to a French student of architecture).

'He is very good at German, but will he be good enough at it when we go to Munich next year?' (French woman).

Up to a certain age, at least, the child is dependent on the parents' decisions and, more particularly, on the place in which one of the parents carries out his or her profession. Thus the parents are able to develop (and sometimes have to develop) carefully thought out education strategies because there are significant differences between the systems and provisions made in each country. It is difficult, for instance, to make a comparison between the educational qualifications of different countries.

A child from a mixed marriage must have a certain level of maturity in order to cope with a mosaic of choices if they are not to get lost in a maze. Here too the child from the upper classes will be at an important advantage, whereas the child from the working classes runs the risk of coming out badly in terms of the choices made on their behalf.

Moreover, depending on each family, choices come at specific points in the life of the couple or of the family. Have the partners been married for only a short time? Their choices will not be so significant while their children are very young. On the other hand, they may be taking on a great responsibility after several years of married life, especially if they have a number of children. The mother's professional activity outside of the home may also have an influence, especially if she lives abroad. She will entrust her child to various social institutions which will develop certain cultural characteristics in keeping with the country in which the family is living. Indeed the place of residence and the socio-professional position of the parents will play a decisive role when it comes to the point of making decisions.

It is also important, however, to take into account the wishes, albeit naive, of the children, since they will be sharing everyday life with friends whose behaviour and choices they will tend to want to adopt. The context of daily life, going to school and making friends are all factors and circumstances which will guide the children in their preferences and decision making. They will form their own bonds with the culture of the country and form their own allegiances, just as they will also reject and keep themselves separate from certain other things in the range of difficult choices that have to be made as they grow up.

**Notes to Chapter 10**

1. *L'Opinion*, Rabat, 27th February 1979.

2. *France Inter*, 23rd February 1979.
3. Émile Durkheim, *Éducation et Sociologie* [Education and Sociology]. Paris: PUF, 1968, p. 41.
4. Erwin Panofsky uses this term in *Achitecture Gothique et Pensée Scolastique*, Minuit edition, Paris 1967, Chapter 2 (translation and postface by Pierre Bourdieu).
5. Jean-Claude Passeron, *Pedagogie et Pouvoir* [Pedagogy and Power], *Encyclopedia Universalis*, Vol. XII, p. 677.
6. SRI (Secretariat for Relations with Islam), 71 Rue de Grenelle, 75007 Paris. This organisation has been inspired for many years by Father Michel Serain.
7. This linguistic term is found above all in the writings of Jean-Paul Sartre.
8. *Études* [Studies], November 1979, pp. 485-507 (Michael Lonsdale interview by Jean Mambrino).

# 11  The independent adolescent

*'I'm not like my cousins'*

## Physical Differences

There was a time when we thought she would walk out on us all. She always loved my father. But I sometimes felt it was very difficult for her. She was homesick and wanted to go back to her own country (Sylvie, aged 18, daughter of a Franco-Norwegian couple).

Her mother had arrived in France just before her marriage at the age of 24. She had left Norway, her homeland, and it was not long before she had three children. The whole family lived in this provincial town where the husband had been born, had all his friends, and was deeply engrossed in his profession.

I have to admit that my father was always out in connection with his work. My mother was kept busy with us. But she often looked very sad (Sylvie).

This was not always the case. She did have a good Swedish friend, also married to a Frenchman. They would very often meet as fellow Scandinavians. The mother had managed to find a balance in her adaptation to a foreign country she was gradually learning more about. Until the day her friend left the country for good, that is. Her husband, a manager in a paper and cardboard company, was being moved within the multinational company which employed him. It had activities in various countries, including France and Sweden.

This had a profound effect on me. I even felt that she was only staying in France for the sake of us, her children.

Sylvie's mother tries to make one or two trips a year to Norway. However, the recent death of her father has reawakened her feeling of homesickness. This had not escaped the notice of her daughter who soon realised that her parents were experiencing a number of problems as a result of being a mixed couple. But she also became aware that children attributed greater significance to these problems.

She had been baptised a Catholic because she lived in this provincial town where her father's devout family would not have liked the fact of her remaining unbaptised or becoming a Protestant, her mother's religion. Having ecumenical leanings, the mother made no objection against this wish.

Whatever decision had been taken would not have made much difference to me. I feel close to my French cousins and see them quite often. It's different with my Norwegian cousins, of course: I only see them once a year when we go on holiday.

The mixed child, in this case the daughter of a Franco-Norwegian couple, is heir to the consequences of her parents' mixed relationship. Can such a child be like the other adolescents of the same age?

Well, I don't feel any great difference when I'm with my friends. It is in the home that I realise we are not like other families. In that sense we are quite unusual . . . For instance, we've always gone to Norway for holidays. It was a regular thing. And we were glad to go there so that we could keep up relations with my mother's family.

She also told me that this was the last year they would be going as a family because she wanted to see something of other countries. She had plans to return to Norway alone so that she could discover it for herself. Looked at from the outside, this family would seem to be like any other family in the neighbourhood. Sylvie's brothers engage in the same activities as their friends do. The parents take turns ferrying them to and from tennis or swimming. Their names (Johan and Mikael), of course distinguish them from other children to a certain extent. But these might easily be Breton names . . . People know that she is a tall, blond Norwegian. But she is treated like any other French woman.

She has been here for over twenty years and there is no difference. We meet her when we go shopping. She often joins in at parents' evenings. She has a slight accent, but that doesn't mean anything (a neighbour).

Nevertheless, this woman had a dual identity. Her eighteen year old daughter is quite aware of this and notices the way in which her mother has to adapt when outside of the home and in contact with French people:

She is quite different with us when we're at home. It's her Norwegian identity which comes to the surface. She sometimes says a few words to us in Norwegian, especially when she is being particularly affectionate with us. I've noticed the same thing when she is angry. At such times, she seems unable to control herself and her true identity comes through. I also noticed it once when she was having a heated discussion with my father.

The child is not taken in, therefore. She is quite able to tell the difference, whatever the neighbours may say. Because she lives within the home, the child is aware that her mother has a secret identity which she is only willing to reveal and express before her husband and children. This young woman had long talks with her mother on the life of women in Scandinavian countries. Although she might outwardly be described as fairly liberated, or as a feminist, she realises from her mother's example that the family and children are very important.

My mother is a bit backward in this respect: she often gives me advice and doesn't want me to be late in. She is also suspicious of French men.

Is this Norwegian woman a special case? Naturally her position as an isolated woman reinforces her maternal instinct which is strongly focused on her children. They become the privileged confidants of an isolated parent. Being far away from her own country, this mother found it quite natural at times to speak to her daughter (and younger sons) as though she were still in Norway:

This often proves quite difficult. My mother does not always realise that the French way is different from the Norwegian way. I notice this when we're on holiday. She reacts to me in the same way as her sisters do to their children.

Sylvie recognises, in her mother's thoughts on education and child rearing, a certain continuity which she would like to transmit. The mixed child may become the object of self-perpetuation on the part of the two societies which claim his allegiance. He or she can become nothing more than a pawn between different ways of thinking and different value systems. The parent 'living in exile' may well have a tendency to be over-attentive to certain aspects of their relationship with the children in order to influence them in favour of his or her own culture. The children will not really be free to make their own choices until gaining independence. Although she has been influenced to a considerable extent by her mother, Sylvie knows that she must be true to both heritages.

In a sense I am in a similar position to my mother. At home I allow the Norwegian part of me to show. There is something of a Norwegian atmosphere in our house. But once we go out, we are in France.

\*\*\*

Her father, my uncle, has a certain authority over me. But my father does not have the same authority over her, though he is her paternal uncle (Saida, aged 22, cousin of Lelia).

I met with these two young women for a whole afternoon at Lelia's parents' home; her father is Tunisian and her mother French. I had dinner with the whole family and had the chance to discuss things with them at length. The parents were in agreement that a married couple has a very important role to play in the education of their children. They did not give in to the pressures exerted by the wider family.

'My mother-in-law would have liked things to be different; so would my brothers-in-law' (Lelia's mother, a French woman, aged 45).

This French woman who had lived in Tunisia for almost twenty years was quite happy with the education she had given her children, in agreement with her husband, and told me that the choice of forenames had been primarily a question of pronunciation. The family goes to France every year on holiday and it is important that her own parents be able to call the children by name without too much difficulty.

At Christmas we make a nativity scene. It is a family display. We don't go to mass. My children are called *infidels* by their Muslim cousins because we don't have any religious belief. They feel themselves to be very different from them. Apart from Lelia who has a good relationship with her cousin. But it is not regarded in a very favourable light by the family. Lelia could have an influence on her cousin who is younger than herself. At the back of it all is me, the foreigner: I am the one they really distrust (as above).

The marriage of this Tunisian, although he was living in his own country, caused a certain breakdown in relationships with his family. He was not actually living in the same town as his parents and all his brothers and sisters. He did not want them to be continually interfering in his family, particularly in the upbringing of his children. Lelia acknowledged that she felt more at ease with her French cousins and had more in common with them. Apart from Saida, she had very little close contact with her Muslim cousins. This young Franco-Tunisian girl is very much at home with her Western-style family life. She has plans to study in France and is eager to retain her French affiliation.

> My father allows me complete freedom to make my own choices. This is made easier by his professional position. He treats boys and girls alike. He doesn't make a distinction. In this respect he is unlike other Tunisian fathers (Lelia).

Her cousin, who took part in our discussion, followed Lelia's opinions and nodded: 'It's not like that with my father. But my mother is Tunisian and I have the whole Tunisian family behind me, or on my back, depending on how you want to look at it'. She pointed out the difference in upbringing, especially if one compares the traditional Muslim family (or 'clan') and Lelia's family (which is much more like the so-called nuclear family living by itself). In some areas there is a real conflict of ideas. The community type of family, with its advantages, constraints and inconveniences, is in competition with the isolated nuclear family in which individual bonds take the form of relationships between one individual and another.

Moreover, the affinity Lelia feels with her French cousins is a real one. However, they only meet during holidays when they are all more available and free to talk than in their everyday lives which are beset with various constraints. Holidays are an excuse for family gatherings and celebrations in which Lelia, her sister and brothers are, to an extent, placed on the *family stage*. Seen only in favourable circumstances, they are welcomed as guests. In France they meet up with a large family which makes a greater expression of its affection in moments of greater intensity than could be the case in the daily pressure of life in Tunisia which they experience with their father's family. Holidays, in this sense, are in sharp contrast with everyday life, but they are at the same time a special time for seeing things in a new light. Lelia expresses this very well. When returning from a parish fête in the middle of August, three years ago, she realised how different her father was.

> He really stood out against all the other people there. Of course he looks a typical N.W. African. I was suddenly confronted by the fact that some people were staring at him.

These country people, firmly rooted in their native soil, were surprised to see a 'foreigner' walking around from one stand to the next. It is true that his southern Tunisian origins gave him strongly pronounced physical characteristics. But Lelia had never been aware of this in Tunisia where they lived. Her father was not different from other men. It was actually her mother who was different. Nevertheless she was fully accepted where she had lived for the last twenty years. This young woman realised for the first time that her father would be a foreigner in France if they had to live there . . .

Another thing came home to her:

As soon as we got back from the fête, I went straight to the bathroom and stood in front of the mirror. It was then that I realised how physically different I was. I had certain features from my father. To that extent I was unlike my cousins. In Tunisia, the question didn't arise. In France, on the other hand, there was this clear difference. What's more, my name was Lelia: I was the only one to have this name. It was impossible for me to go unnoticed. People were looking at me too. Later on, when we went to the Lafayette Gallery, I had the impression that people recognised that I was of N.W. African origin.

It was on this occasion that she came face to face with her uncertain identity, her double allegiance. She now felt more at home when with her friends at the lycée in Tunis than among the girls her cousins had introduced her to when she was on holiday. But she was not particularly close to her Tunisian cousins either. On a number of occasions she had had heated discussions with them on the role of women. They were strongly opposed to her feminist arguments. The only close relationship she had was with her cousin Saida; she had nothing at all in common with her other Tunisian female cousins whom she only met at the big Muslim festivals in Southern Tunisia where large family gatherings are the custom.

'I feel no link with the future of my children. They will leave us in any case' (Lelia's mother).

I confronted the mother with the possibility of leaving Tunisia. She explained that it would be difficult for her daughter to settle and marry in Tunisia. Her critical spirit, her liking for lively discussion meant that she would be regarded as unmarriageable:

It seems to me that the family in Tunisia has always developed in the context of marriage and not in the context of love. Marriage here is thought of as a contract of duties and obligations. What is more, people speak of a marriage contract here, rather than of a marriage certificate (Lelia's mother).

Lelia was indeed influenced by the concept of marriage for love. She would not allow a choice to be made for her. Her father was quite aware

of this and was quite in agreement with her, which is understandable in
that he had not even married within his own group. By the strength of his
personality and through persuasion, he had managed to overcome a
number of difficulties and areas of opposition.

I will always give my children their freedom; after all, I took this
freedom for myself at a certain point in my life. And it was very costly.
But they must also learn that freedom always involves risks and taking
responsibility for one's own actions (Lelia's father).

***

There are many points of difference between Sylvie and Lelia which
have to do primarily with where they actually live. Sylvie feels quite at
home in her environment. She feels that she belongs, at home in her home
town, in the area where she lives, and with her friends. Lelia also lives in
the country where she was born, but she has been strongly influenced by
her mother's western culture. She sometimes feels alienated. Feeling
attracted by France, where she has only ever been when on holiday, she
has many questions about her future. She is already aware of a number
of problems connected with remaining in her father's country. She is happy
about coming back when she has spent some time, however short, in
France. Sylvie has no problems of this type. Norway remains a foreign
country to her. She is fully French and has no intentions of living in
Norway, and certainly not of marrying a foreigner. She has seen too much
of the pain her mother has suffered in isolation because of Sylvie and her
brothers. Lelia's mother, on the other hand, has embraced the Tunisian
way of life; she has taken courses in Arabic and now speaks it fluently.
She has a great deal of contact with Tunisians, as well as with French
women. She is a member of an informal group of French women, most
of whom are married to N.W. African men. When they get together they
talk about their respective situations, both in the home and in society.
Their main concern, of course, is the quality of their integration into
Tunisian society without at the same time losing their French identity.

Both Sylvie and Lelia are from privileged classes, free from the
worries which can loom so large in mixed homes of more modest means.
Lelia is less of a foreigner in France than a girl of the same age from an
immigrant family, living in a run-down inner city area. The child from a
mixed marriage most certainly has a personal journey to make; but it is
often similar to the journey which has to be made by the child of parents
of the same nationality. However, the child from a mixed family often has
to make choices which other children do not encounter. There are some
extraordinary journeys which are not often the privilege of children from

mixed families. One example of this is the child of a Franco-Muslim couple who, after a long period of heart searching, became a priest.

*** 

There are many examples of children from Judeo-Christian couples who experience gripping, though often very painful, lives. One such couple had three children: a young man aged nineteen, a daughter of seventeen and a boy of fifteen. When the mother left Strasbourg to study in Paris, she met Robert who was taking a degree course in biology. She was immediately attracted to him because of his romantic, musical nature. He was dark with black eyes. She was gripped by the story of his life and that of his parents. His father had had to leave Poland at the time of the pogroms. He escaped as a refugee to France and, without knowing a word of the language, very soon married a practicing Catholic against everyone's advice. The family had gone through many difficulties; only one brother and one sister had managed to escape with him. All three of them were now settled in France, married to French partners.

Robert had very clear memories of that period in the past, and of his half-Jewish/half-Christian childhood. I met him two days after the attack on the Rue Copernic synagogue in Paris in 1980. 'Why do they still hold so much against us?' he asked me. I pointed out that he had used the word 'us': what did he mean by that?

At times like these I feel myself to be very Jewish. It's a question of allegiance to what I must admit is sometimes a mythical community. Although she understands me, Claire cannot fully share this with me. It is all bound up with the history of my father's family, and with the experiences of my parents during the war. My mother is a practising Catholic who has never missed mass. I now realise what courage she showed in doing what she did at that time. She had to face rejection by her whole family. None of her friends wanted anything more to do with her. She had sided with the Jews. She is still an active supporter of the MRAP[1]. She knows from first-hand experience both the downright stupidity as well as the logical points of racism.

This was the first of a series of discussions in which I got to know this man. Robert was an attractive person. His identity as the son of a Judeo-Christian marriage did not bother him unduly. He was not prone to nostalgia. He knew, however, that his past had been a disturbed one. His children, who were now grown up, asked him many questions which he answered quite frankly. They learned that, during the last war, their father's parents who were living in Paris at the time would weep as they listened to the radio pouring out vile nonsense about the Jews, blaming them for all the ills which France was suffering. The cowardliness of the Vichy government, the compromising on the part of the high officials aligned them at once with the Resistance movement instigated by General de Gaulle. Robert remembers his uncle being involved in the underground movement. They did not speak about it much at home because it had to be kept a secret. The commissariat for Jewish affairs may have been instrumental in providing information against certain Jews. His father often exploded in response to the overtly racist remarks he heard on the radio: 'What are they trying to do to us? Will France also become a country that people need to flee from?'

It was then that Robert realised that there was an important difference between himself and his classmates. Did he not hear such words as Yid and Jewboy in the playground? The teacher, however, with some caution of course, would reprove the pupils: 'You are here to learn, not to show contempt'. He went through a period of great tension in his family at that time which helped him to endure a great number of things. It seemed as though two opposing worlds were existing alongside one another. The world outside of the home, in the street and at school with classmates, gave him the feeling of being completely French. He was actually playing a part in order that no one would guess that there was any Jewish blood in him. The other world was the inner one: the home where, through his father, he learned that he was one with and belonged to the group of people who were being treated with contempt and hounded.

A new anxiety was aroused in me. I wasn't after all just like my cousins on my mother's side. I even wondered on one occasion whether my cousins at X were themselves racist as far as Jews were concerned. I saw so little of them. My father was not particularly accepted in the wider Catholic family of my mother.

He knew that there was something Jewish within him. Especially when he went to see his father's sister who had married a fellow Jew and kept all the traditions.

I can still smell the cakes she made for the traditional festivals and remember what they tasted like. I still like unleavened bread and can't get enough of it.

At one time, Robert told me, he felt that he had a special mission. By hiding his Jewishness, he was wanting to show his class superiority and applied himself to doing well in his studies, homework and lessons.

That's what it came down to. Later on I realised that I was doing all this in order to look good, so that no one would have anything to find fault with in me. This is very Jewish, this desire to demonstrate various good qualities to the outside world. It should be remembered that the Jews were being blamed with all sorts of defects ... It was important to make a good show. One could not be both Jewish and mediocre.

A great process of development was taking place in this young child's personality. His father was quite proud of this. His sister Isabelle was also to do well later on. But she experienced less hostility than her brother in her peaceful primary school for girls. In an environment where only boys are together, mischievous violence can sometimes be quite traumatic. Robert remembers one painful incident in his class when he was barely ten years old. A group of tough classmates imposed their own system of law on others not belonging to their group, intimidating the younger ones in the playground. Why were they so hard on Vincent Mermann, a small child a year younger than the rest of them, who was a brilliant pupil? Was it just jealousy? Or were they being affected by the climate of opinion in France, and in their families, at that time? 'Vincent is a Jew, Vincent is a Jew', they started singing at the end of one break time. The teacher immediately silenced them. Later on, however, Vincent was dragged from the playground to the toilets and told to let down his trousers. 'We want to see your penis'. He could do nothing to protect himself from the physical force of the four bigger children who were holding him and already hurting him. 'We know you're a Jew and trying to hide it'. The whole school heard about this. The news was whispered throughout the school. These bullies had caused a serious problem. Vincent never came back to school. The incident was very worrying for Robert who, throughout the affair, retained a neutrality which made him feel uneasy ... What about him? He had not been circumcised, of course, thanks to his mother who had had him baptised into the Catholic religion. He nevertheless felt an inner sense of solidarity with this Vincent whom he was never to see again.

From that point on he realised that his life would always be characterised by a certain ambiguity. It would be difficult for him to feel he belonged anywhere because of the choices made earlier by his parents.

I certainly feel it is better for parents to make some sort of choice than to leave the child in a complete vacuum ... saying that the child can choose for himself when he is older.

Robert recalled his own life, his own personal journey. He affirmed that it was easier to make decisions on the basis of choices already taken in the past than to make a random choice in a void. Many children from Judeo-Christian families have later chosen the religion they felt more at home in, thus rejecting or confirming the original choice made by their parents.

This strong feeling of dual allegiance became increasingly important to Robert as he continued with his education. Particularly when he started on his philosophy course and read the great authors. Was he not also interested in Brittany, his mother's birth place, and Poland where his father was born? Belonging to two different groups did not mean belonging half to one group and half to another. He realised that he needed to break new ground in two places at the same time. Eventually, he was able to establish two sets of roots. He had to admit, however, that this was made much easier by the fact that he was living in Paris.

The war period left Robert with painful feelings of cowardliness and shame. To begin with people did not really understand what was going on. But he saw the yellow stars. This came as a great shock to him. He imagined how passers-by would look at his father.

On one occasion I believe there was something going on between my mother and father; there was some sort of argument. My father, on edge because of the position of Jews, was unable to express his disapproval openly. He tended to take full advantage of my mother's patience. She must sometimes have imagined him wearing a yellow star. But my mother was unable to think such a thing. I was wrong. Tolerance had become the rule for her life.

This child saw his parents in a situation in which external conflicts were threatening to upset their marriage. So they tended to withdraw from society and become a close-knit family unit. Threatened by aggression from outside, Robert, Isabelle his sister, and his parents formed a very close group. For a long time afterwards they retained this sense of closeness. 'We were not at all like the others, and needed to protect ourselves'. Robert thought of his parents' identity. The remarks he heard about Jews, and the reading of certain newspapers — particularly *Le Pilori* — shocked him deeply. He gradually developed a hard shell so that he would no longer hear what was being said. These malicious attacks were aimed at the image of the father whom he loved. He was already siding with his Jewish father.

It was very difficult for him to choose which camp he belonged to, for he was neither choosing to be a Jew nor to be a non-Jew. He rejected this distinction. He adopted the concise formula of Isabelle, his far less intellectual sister: 'You love them . . . You are Robert. Full stop'. He nevertheless felt a sense of solidarity with the one who was under attack. Had he not learned in catechism classes that Jesus was always on the side of the rejected and the ill-treated? Did he not have some of his father's Jewish features? There was no doubt in Isabelle's case: she was pretty in a 'universal' sense. He, on the other hand, was beginning to wonder whether his dark hair and eyes might become an embarrassing pointer to his origins. 'Don't be so silly. Mum is dark and has black eyes as well. You just take after her', Isabelle had said. He felt reassured. But he also appreciated the gross stupidity of some ideologies which had drawn typical Jewish portraits. By doing so, they had isolated certain racial characteristics, and caused those who had them to end up hating themselves.

Robert liked traditional Jewish music. Through the years he had collected a number of records he enjoyed listening to. He was not a practising Jew, of course. The main festivals were enough for him. It was his aunt, more than anyone else, who encouraged such observances, inviting all the family to take part. She would immerse the whole world around her in what she called a 'Jewish bath'. But he had also often attended mass with his mother who is very committed to her faith. Indeed, a Dominican father, who had become a friend of the whole family, would often come to dinner. Robert welcomed his visits because he did not attempt to convert anyone and was very tolerant.

Yet he had a number of stories to tell about his dealings with Catholicism. From time to time, when he and Isabelle were young, they would visit his mother's family at X in Brittany. Everything was fine during the week. They played happily together with friends and a whole host of cousins. They went catching eels, and had marvellous walks in the forest. But when Sunday came, there was the delicate problem of mass. His mother then felt very divided. So as not to shock the grandparents and her brothers and sisters, who were all committed to their religious observance, she made her children go along. 'It will please Granny'. In that large, cold church they would listen to the readings and to the singing of the skilful parish choir. It was with great awkwardness, however, that they made the sign of the cross. This did not go unnoticed. Their grandmother asked their mother about what religious education they were receiving. For some months they had been attending catechism classes, but somewhat sporadically. They stood out most from their cousins in the fact that they were not communicants. This problem over mass every Sunday always sparked off discussions with the uncles and aunts. Their father always chose to steer clear of these. He had no intention of engaging in a battle which would be lost from the outset.

I have often had the impression that my father adopted a minority attitude to the situation and that he took the course of least possible risk in the face of an ever stronger majority, even if it was wrong.

He once went to midnight mass because he liked it and because Jesus was always a Jew like other Jews in his eyes. Thus Robert and his sister were sometimes involved in situations where they 'had to be all things to all people'. But they would never tolerate racist allusions or 'Jewish stories'. They quickly learned that their father was a *Yid* . . .

I didn't understand what this word meant when I first heard it. I looked in the dictionary and actually found it. From that point on, I felt able to excuse my classmates to an extent, for *Yid* was an official entry in the dictionary, so they were entitled to use it. A dictionary, too, can be racist. However, when my classmates used the word, there was a particular intonation in their voices.

Robert told me how his curiosity had led him to find all the words used in referring to Jews; it was a painful discovery. A whole arsenal of names had been coined over the ages. He discovered such terms as Jewboy, Yid and sheeny. He was surprised, in contrast to this, not to find an entry for *Ravensbrück*, the Nazi concentration camp for women and children. The same dictionary contained a surplus of definitions but there were also glaring omissions. In addition to this, certain factual truths were disguised. Max Jacob, for instance, was shown to have died in Drancy; but there was no mention of the fact that it occurred during internment.

What is quite upsetting is the fact that this dictionary was printed well after the war. How can you fight against racist ideas when they are officially recorded in people's memories?

When the war ended Robert told everyone he knew that he was the son of a Jew. By then people had learned something about the extermination camps, and about Oradour-sur-Glane, the little village razed to the ground by the Nazis on 10th June 1944, killing every man, woman and child. A certain reconciliation then took place with some members of his mother's family. Robert continued his education at a lycée and became a teenager like any other. He became more conscious of his own identity. 'I was becoming more French each day'. His father would always speak to him about Poland, but for Robert, France, or more precisely Paris, was his homeland. The Jewish part of his identity resurfaced whenever he went back to see his mother's family. In Paris, on the other hand, it lay dormant and no one would remark on it. Whereas in this small village near X, he felt different. People knew that Claire's son was half Christian, half Jewish. This had consequences he had not foreseen.

One summer when on holiday, he and his cousins met up with a group of young people. He began to get to know them all, especially Jocelyne whom he liked a lot. She was the daughter of highly respected shopkeepers in the town and often served customers during her holidays. She was a student, and Robert noticed her because of her voice and her blue eyes. He was attracted by her easy-going nature and her frank way of speaking. It took him two weeks to approach her. One day, when they were alone, he spoke to her about *L'Étranger* [The Outsider] by Albert Camus, which had just been published. Robert was feeling very happy and asked Jocelyne if he might hold her hand as they continued their walk alone along the beach. The young woman burst out laughing. It was neither mockery nor consent. She admitted that she had known for some time who he was, not wishing to be racist, but that her parents, ardent followers of Petain, had a hatred she could not understand for the Jews, and she did not want to hurt them. Robert then realised that it had all been wishful thinking.

He learned his lesson from this holiday and from Jocelyne's polite refusal. Behind her words was the social anxiety about what people will think, and she was too afraid to challenge it. To go out with Robert would be to compromise herself with the son of a Pole, and a Jew into the bargain. She would be upsetting a social order which seemed unchangeable. Of course the Jews had suffered during the war, but one did not want to actually form alliances with them. That would be carrying things too far . . .

In Paris Robert met other girls. It was easier there and family pressures were not so intense. He became increasingly more aware of his identity. Was it not with a certain pride that he could one day write: 'Like Proust and Montaigne, I am a half-Jew'?

In a student cafeteria in the Fourteenth district of the city he made the acquaintance of Claire whose parents lived in Z where her father was a tax inspector. They got into the habit of eating at the same table. She was very quiet and 'private', confiding in him that she liked Paris very much. She had no roots because her father had to continually move as he was promoted in his work. She had already lived in Grenoble and Lille. They lived together for some months and then married, quietly, at the Town Hall because Claire very soon became pregnant. It was a very simple ceremony. It was mainly student friends in addition to their families. Claire's father was nothing like the ideas people sometimes have about tax inspectors. He had been on the side of the resistance in the war and acknowledged his anti-racist convictions. He immediately got on with Robert's father, the Jew from Poland. The war was now a thing of the past . . .

\*\*\*

Robert's story, though not perhaps altogether typical, brings out a number of characteristic factors. The child born from a mixed marriage will at times be confronted with unusual situations in what is otherwise a fairly normal environment. These may affect him in the deepest part of his personality. Robert, for instance, had to find a position between the circumcised and the uncircumcised. He now realises that this is of no importance to him. But it troubled him for many years. The desire to form certain contacts often came up against social pressures or deep-rooted prejudices. All these reactions taught him to find his own place in a world where anyone who is not quite like other people is quickly made to feel different. It was only when he became an adult that Robert was able to take a more objective view of events which had loomed larger than life in his childhood and adolescence.

Sylvie, the daughter of the Franco-Norwegian couple, and Lelia, the daughter of the Franco-Tunisian couple, will no doubt have different personal journeys to make in life. They are now going through the experiences of youth and will eventually find more or less appropriate solutions . . . Indeed, depending on where they live and on their age, the children from mixed marriages go through a number of situations with varying degrees of sensitivity. Not all children from mixed marriages live in a favourable family environment which will help them to grow up with a sense of balance.

We can take Karim and his five brothers and sisters as an example. Their mother, who grew up in the care of the local authority, served in a Lyon bar. She married an Algerian from Aures. When Algeria became independent in 1962, the whole family went back to live in the town of Aures. The children were more like their mother in appearance; but they have become completely assimilated into the Auresian people. Their mother has got used the way women live there. She speaks their language. She does not stand out . . . All the children speak the language of the country very well; they are not now so good at French which they were later to learn at school alongside other Auresian children. Since they left France, they have never been back. Where could they go, since their mother does not have any family? They cannot be compared with French children. France is a country which is becoming more and more distant in their memories. They now feel completely Algerian. Becoming rooted in a given culture has undoubtedly become their chance of survival.

\*\*\*

Irene is the daughter of a Polish father and a Breton mother. She has recently married a Breton and her son has a Breton forename. She has only been to Poland once. She regards France as her homeland.

Myriam, the daughter of the man from Kabylia, is completely integrated into the French way of life. She goes back to Algiers every year, but cannot stand the way women are treated there. She is very opposed to the macho image assumed by some men and related certain events which took place in France, in a completely western context. She has just married a Mexican artist whom she met in Paris. 'I'm really a Parisian'.

Isabella goes to the Abruzzi region every year for her holidays. This enables her to visit the large family of her Italian father who has now lived in France for more than twenty-five years.

I'm Italian for one month a year because I speak the language and find it a very enriching experience. But as soon as I'm back in France I feel French again. There is no tension between the two. It is just something I've got used to. I've been going back to my father's village since I was three years old.

Isabella is a blonde with grey-green eyes. She looks just like her student friends.

This is not the case with Vincent whose father is from Gabon.

Because of my halfcaste appearance, I can't disguise my identity. People often think I'm from Martinique. I go to visit my father in Gabon every other year. But I feel most at home in France. I was born here and this is where all my friends are.

Vincent's physical characteristics distinguish him from other children. He is sometimes on the receiving end of racist attitudes. Just because of his appearance. He frequently visits the West Indian areas of Bordeaux. He goes to the annual carnival. He is going out with a girl from Guadeloupe. His mother was divorced more than ten years ago and says: 'I've never been able to remarry; society never forgives you for straying from the path!' It caused a scandal in the village she came from when people saw her going out with a black man. Vincent knows all about this. His maternal grandmother is his main confidante. He is able to tell her most things. But apart from her, he feels somewhat cut off.

The importance of this physical difference increases in certain situations. It is an effective factor for discrimination. Vincent often finds himself being stopped by the police.

I know why: it's my West Indian head they notice. They don't stop other people of my age and height whose hair isn't curly like mine.

The adolescent child of a mixed marriage becomes aware of all these nuances in people's attitudes and he must be constantly 'negotiating' with an environment which may reject, tolerate or single him out. Being physically different is seen straight away as a deviation from the norm. The child therefore has to get over the hurdle of rejection, because there is a whole hierarchy of discriminating factors.

It is mainly the colour difference, depending on how dark a person's skin is; this marks a person out as belonging to a certain group. This is followed by curly hair and the shape of the lips, even if the skin is not dark. Finally, there is the question of the voice or accent which will indicate that a person does not belong to the group of people who speak the language 'correctly'.

When I go out with a girl there's always the moment when she looks at the palms of my hands to see whether they are lighter in colour than the rest of my body. I won't mention other parts of my anatomy. Some girls seem to experience both an attraction and a repulsion at the same time. It's something that has to be lived with (Nicholas, aged 23, son of a Belgian mother and a Congolese father).

Some of these children get on quite well with their physical differences. They even manage to take a certain symbolic advantage of them. When Yannick Noah, the French tennis champion, embraces his Cameroonian father in front of the television cameras at the end of a match, everyone forgets his dark skin. He is admired for his skill at tennis. Noah derives a symbolic advantage from this. This is not the case for a West Indian worker who is stopped on the Metro because of the colour of his skin. In his case the fact that his skin is of a different colour is a disadvantage. It just creates problems for him.

On the basis of these distinguishing characteristics of appearance or the sound of a foreign name, society sets up its hierarchy of acceptability, and rejects those who do not meet its requirements. Is it not the same for handicapped people? In a holiday village in the Massif Central a young Frenchman was unable to find a girl willing to dance with him at a function organised by the management. The reason was that he is an albino.

\*\*\*

The children from a mixed marriage will be put in situations where they take part in the main choices of life. These will involve varying degrees of tension. The parents will already have taken some choices anyway. Sometimes, however, they will have refrained so as to 'leave them greater freedom later on'. These first choices (or the absence of choices) more often than not relate to religious affiliation — Christian baptism or circumcision in the case of Muslims — and nationality. Also involved is the preference for a particular language at a given point in childhood, and the choice of education system and the school the children will attend. These choices or groups of choices are sociological in nature because they are more or less imposed by real-life situations. The temporary or permanent place of residence of the parents imposes a lifestyle and a socio-cultural environment from which it will be difficult for the children to separate themselves. These decisions are taken when the children are young; as the children reach teenage years and become adolescent they will acquire a certain amount of freedom to make their own choices which will result in the rejection, abandoning or embracing of a given social group and culture. They will sometimes have to balance difficulties and ambiguities, if not suffering, with the desire for integration and the achieving of certain plans. It is possible that the course of their education will be based on the profession chosen in light of their future in one country or another. Then there is the question of military service which will result in the acquisition of a nationality.

The legal hurdle of eighteen years of age will require thought about the choices which adolescents would rather put off. They may blame their parents for not having accepted their responsibilities. They may think that the decisions would have been easier to make if they had been taken for them when they were still children. These pre-choices, or provisional choices, would have been a basis for making other decisions. They might have preferred this to having everything left to have to decide as they grew up.

'When he is older, he can decide for himself', many parents say. This is often just a smoke-screen to hide a certain embarrassment and a desire to evade responsibility as mixed parents. Society will instead impose its own choices. The child will then find him or herself fully integrated into the French way of life as a result of having received all their education in France, despite the fact of having always been told that they also have another nationality. When choices are deferred until the child is able to decide for themself, this often leaves the child in an impossible situation, unable to exercise this new freedom. Earlier choices made by the parents would have been a basis for discussion of other choices. It might happen that the child questions the whole of his past, but at least they will be able to do so consciously.

Children certainly pose complex problems for mixed couples and these are difficult to get out of. Children oblige the parents to be aware of the significance of their actions. Their choices should be in harmony with the needs, for they will be immediately followed by certain consequences. The children may blame them at certain times, for ambiguous decisions when they would have preferred them to take clear-cut decisions. The child of a divorced mixed couple may suffer serious personal damage as the result of the parents' disagreement, but may also — in this critical situation — become the victim of vague decision making on his or her behalf in the past.

If the bond between the parents is broken, the child will quickly become a pawn between two individuals, and considered as their property, over whom they will feel entitled to exercise the prerogative of choice. Each will want to make all the decisions. The child can even become an instrument of blackmail between two societies. Because the parents were unable to make the necessary parental and emotional choices, it will be left up to courts to decide in their place, at a dramatic time in the child's life.

It is not therefore astonishing that painful stories often appear in the press in connection with abducted or kidnapped children. 'I am hiding my daughter', one mother told me. She is afraid that her husband will carry out his threat to abduct their child to whom he only has access during holidays. Must a child left in a no-man's land between two societies choose to live with one parent while they are in the process of getting divorced? The child might also get the impression of choosing one parent in preference to the other. Instead of allowing things to develop to such a critical state, the parents should have adopted a philosophy of choices, as a means of becoming integrated into society, in order to enable the child to become familiarised with the environment in which he or she will eventually come to terms with an independent way of life, particularly with respect to the possible ups and downs in the parents' relationship.

Do the children from a mixed marriage simply have half of two different identities? Are they half-French and half something else? Or do they instead become the dynamic synthesis of a dual cultural allegiance made up of elements which, as they combine, enhance both cultures by bringing them together in a positive way?

## Notes to Chapter 11

1. Mouvement Contre le Racisme et Pour l'Amitié Entre les Peuples.

# Part 4
# Hopes and Realities

# 12 Separation and divorce

*'I feel guilty about the children'*

Many mixed marriages end in divorce. And why should this not be the case? It just shows that Love with a capital L is not always enough for 'those who were once strangers to one another ... '. If marriages really did last on the basis of Love, there would hardly be any divorce. Social reality teaches us quite the opposite. Divorce is rife in all areas especially in mixed couples.

The partners in a mixed marriage do not have any time in which misunderstandings can accumulate. They crop up all too quickly and take root surreptitiously, as they do in non-mixed marriages. If the partners are not watchful at difficult times, certain words and expressions can soon create an irreversible, irredeemable situation. It is sometimes too much to require that a husband and wife, who are already separated naturally by their 'foreignness', somehow reduce the distance that they have allowed to develop between them. A breakdown has occurred and it is no longer possible to 'link up the carriages'. This situation inevitably leads to divorce.

In the face of an environment which may have been very hostile to their marriage the success of a couple's relationship becomes the objective of the partners in their attempt to prove that they were right in choosing to get married so that no one will have anything to blame them for. A high price has to be paid for this quest for harmony. It is brought about at the cost of a *sustained effort*, particularly for the foreign partner. The latter is called upon to demonstrate his or her qualities as a marriage partner and the ability to become integrated into the other partner's community. The foreign wife will have to do her utmost to live up to the standards for wives as laid down by the dominant society, not to mention the standards expected of mothers and possibly also of working women. She will be presented with roles and images, and be expected to live up to them. At the level of the couple themselves the husband may consciously or unconsciously expect his wife to live up to his expectations which may sometimes be unrealistic given their situation.

How is the marriage knot untied? Official divorce is actually a purely legal measurement, and many non-mixed couples do not make their separation official in the form of a divorce. The practice of living parallel lives, side by side, can become a tacit agreement, allowing a couple to *stay together without living together*. In the case of the mixed couple, however, the more or less conscious level of expectations of the partners will not stand up to this form of separation which might otherwise seem a convenient solution. Too much is at stake in a mixed relationship for it to be possible for one partner to be allowed to dominate the situation, e.g. with respect to the children's education.

A couple's integration into a given environment is often fraught with difficulties, and these may be to a greater extent loaded against the foreign partner. Much has been required of him or her. The foreign partner has had to make a great personal investment in the marriage. Divorce may then be perceived as an act of dispossession as though some fraud had been committed. After having first consented to being converted to a new way of life, the foreign partner feels deeply wounded by his or her mistake. A social outcast from his original group which has been left behind, he or she has now spoilt the chance of acceptance by the newly chosen environment in which it will be difficult to succeed alone.

What saddens me most of all in this matter of divorce is that I would have found it impossible to imagine this happening only three months ago. I am becoming more and more racist (African, aged 25, about to get divorced).

Divorce in a mixed couple will be determined by their social position in the country, and the degree to which their relationship is a mixed one will often only serve to aggravate the situation. A husband and wife who are both doctors will tend to have a more privileged lifestyle which will enable them to take a more detached view of certain difficulties. A working class couple, on the other hand, will experience severe restraints on their lives on top of the fact that they are mixed, which will make this even more difficult and painful to bear.

Does the fact that one of the partners is a foreigner make it more difficult for them to resolve conflicts than if they were both of the same nationality? Yes and no. A mixed couple will nevertheless be particularly sensitive to any break-up, simply because of the objective differences which the partners will not always be able to reduce:

I am the French woman and my husband is 'the American': that's how they refer to him around here (French woman, aged 36, married to an American).

An unremitting quest to discount any patently obvious differences can have side-effects on the foreign partner who may feel standardised, naturalised or brought into line. This is the path of false identity which may be hard to bear.

Many people do not feel at home in their skin, because it is not their own[1] (Émile Ajar).

There are impenetrable barriers to the system of mutual concessions, because the pressure from society often overrides their personal desires to ignore it completely. In one Franco-American couple the Anglo-Saxon identity of the husband is accepted by the French wife and there is no question of the husband's being required to give up that identity. In another couple, the French wife, an office worker, always made efforts to hide the fact that she had a mixed marriage, keeping secret the identity of her Moroccan husband, a law student.

You're more French than I am. It's only perhaps when we're alone together that your Arab side comes out.

He was very attracted to this woman right from the beginning. But they were later to go through various crises and experience bitter attitudes which led them to divorce despite having two children. They were unable to achieve a balance and to accept the fact that they were mixed. She too was attracted to him: she liked this Moroccan student's physique and appreciated his 'kindness, care, gentleness and affection'. But she could not bring herself to accept his family, his true identity and his Islamic origins, although he did not practise his religion. Little by little two different types of behaviour developed in this marriage. The husband became closer to his colleagues and friends by suppressing his Moroccan identity more and more; at the same time this identity became increasingly more apparent to his wife, though he never displayed it outside of the home. His wife could not put up with these two very contradictory ways of behaving because she wanted to see him become like every other Frenchman, since he was not really like the average Arab. Finding it impossible to get on with one another, they decided to separate so that they could have time to think. Since she did not have a job, the woman took her children to stay with her parents in another town. While continuing his studies he took a job because his grant was not enough for running two homes. He too ended up going back to his family for a while in Morocco.

The *separating function* of separation had its effect.When they met again they had nothing further they wanted to say to one another, apart from settling some financial matters and deciding on how the children were to be cared for. It was then only necessary for them to make some joint plans which had to do with the children and where they would live. He then went off to do some serious work in a company in Paris for a few months. She resumed her studies which had been interrupted. It only took one year for divorce to be pronounced and the man went back to his home land where he married a Moroccan woman. Each of them returned to their original cultures where they found their original identities.

Can the above divorce be attributed to the mere fact that they were a mixed couple? It may have had something to do with it, but is probably not the only reason for the break-up of their relationship. As shown by L. Roussel[2] the development of traditional marriage in general terms towards a type of marriage/companionship relationship involves a greater instability in marriages in that it has to do with the choice of a partner who is becoming increasingly more isolated from the original social context. Mixed marriage is precisely this type of union in which the choice is made outside of the group as a deliberate act — i.e. free from all restraints — of one individual who assumes all responsibility for that choice. For a couple like this, marriage has in no way been arranged by the families. It may often have been disapproved of by the families. The partners had no prior common interests or property to safeguard. We are not thinking here of some royal marriages, of course, or marriages between extremely wealthy people who, in coming together, pool vast resources and interests.

The latest figures on the number of divorces show a significant development in several countries. In 1960 there was one divorce for each four marriages in France.[3] It is difficult to isolate the figures for mixed marriages but these will certainly have followed the general trend. After all, mixed marriage is even more exposed to the unfulfilled expectations of each partner.

Taking France as an example, and linked with industrialisation and urbanisation, and to the change from a rural to an urban country, the development of divorce has followed that of the family in its progression from the enlarged family to the nuclear family that we see today. Divorce is more frequent in large urban areas, particularly when the parents do not have any financial interests in common — e.g. land — in the country. Alternatively, these interests may have lost their importance once the partners are settled in the town as wage earners, except where the couple work together as shopkeepers for then there may be certain distinct advantages in staying together.

Indeed, throughout the French population such couples tend to divorce less than any other profession, whereas mixed marriages may, in one way, be 'predestined' for divorce more frequently than is the case with other marriages. Most of such couples tend to live in towns and have little or no property of their own — at least in the first years of their marriage. Moreover they do not have a family line to continue. We have already seen how, in marrying outside of the group, this type of couple has also to a certain extent placed itself outside of the circle of interests which could preserve, maintain and pass on the group interests to its members.

The partners of marriages which have broken up will experience divorce in different ways. Some people take a fairly philosophical view of it. 'We got divorced with a certain amount of regret, but we just couldn't live together any more. It got to the point where my most precious experiences were about to be obliterated'. A breakdown in a mixed couple's (and very often in a non-mixed couple's) relationship is not the failure of the couple's whole life together, but of just a certain part. The couple may have been happy, living in harmony for several years, and this separation may simply be the realisation that they cannot go any further. They are unable, or unwilling, to venture on a new lap which may seem difficult to them.

In any case I do not regret anything I did and I would do it again. Perhaps not in the same circumstances (. . .). I certainly didn't waste my time. Having said that, of course, I do feel somewhat guilty about the children . . . They don't have their father around any more and that's important for children (French woman, aged 31, divorced with three children).

In the eyes of the social group as a whole, certain reservations and arguments were raised when the couple first came together. Some divorced partners will tend to justify themselves before that same social group. They do not want to lose face in any sense. They place some of the blame on their family's lack of understanding at the start of their marriage with the foreigner. 'My family did nothing to support us or to help my ex-husband become integrated into our society'. This woman is recalling the time when her parents made an unannounced visit to Paris to see what sort of 'head' her partner had. 'Good, that's all right, he doesn't have an Arab head', her mother said to her; her father reproached her for not living with someone of the same educational level as herself.

'They just came to see whether he was presentable'. In fact, though he was 'acceptable', this man from Kabylia was never actually accepted by the woman's family.

Firstly, this woman is attributing part of the blame for her divorce on her family 'who had never understood her since she was a child'. Secondly, she recognises that she had too idealised a picture of marriage from the moment she first met her fiancé. They wanted to love 'above their means', without taking account of what was actually possible:

> I can now understand how difficult it is for someone who has never found their own balance in life and then tries to find it in marriage (. . .). I don't think this has anything to do with whether or not the marriage is mixed.

What part did the fact that this marriage was mixed have to play in the subsequent divorce? Perhaps one might ask another question: was not the very fact that this marriage was mixed attributable to the individuals who were already predestined or socially disposed towards certain types of behaviour and certain acts which would leave them somewhat apart from the general standards of their social group? Mixed marriage, or an encounter with a foreigner, is one of these behaviour patterns which, not being subject to the normal restraints, places the individuals outside of, or at the edge of, the group. It may be in keeping with previous conduct, unless of course contracting a mixed marriage takes the form of a sudden break and withdrawal from the social group. Indeed, divorce and mixed marriage are nothing more than the logical outworking of some individuals' personalities in cases where those individuals wanted to create a real separation between themselves and the other members of the group. As E. Durkheim says, there are often social parallels between two distinct phenomena. Divorce is just the final stage of a mixed relationship (not its objective consequence), one more stage, the logical and chronological sequel in the life of certain individuals. Marriage was the previous stage which may, in turn, have been preceded by a time spent in a foreign country, one stage among others which adorn the biographical course followed and the personal journey through life. What happened before the foreign partner was encountered may well have been the cause both of the mixed marriage and of the eventual divorce. Here too we see parallel consequences which can be traced back to the same origins.

Moreover, the social differences between the partners in a mixed marriage may be more important than religious and cultural differences. In the case of a couple consisting of a French woman school teacher and a N.W. African skilled worker, the social difference between them will be greater than the actual cultural difference. The social situation of each partner will produce points of view based on their respective social positions, and these points of view will be superimposed on their cultural and religious positions. Each will thus have a value and reference system. The divergence of the systems of the two partners can be a source of tension which invades all areas of their married life. The partners may have tried to reduce the cultural gap without having done enough to deal with the social gap which is also an indication of their objective personalities (in contrast with their subjective personalities which they endeavour to show to one another). Divorce is more prevalent in France between partners who are very different in terms of social and geographic background.

Since mixed couples will have a greater number of areas of difference, the relationship will be that much more fragile. Rather than having an accumulative effect, these additional differences have a multiplying effect.

The fact of not being born in the same country, for instance, often involves differences of religion and culture. A man from a Catholic farming family in Brittany is very different from his wife who is from a middle-class family in Stockholm. She is blonde and taller than her husband who has brown hair and a sturdy physique. Moreover, if she is fairly lax about religious observance (she is a Protestant), she will not always be prepared for her children to go to mass regularly on Sundays with her husband's parents who do not live far away. The simple fact of geographic distance in this case also involves cultural differences which are highlighted even more by the difference in social status. The husband cannot, due to his allegiances, 'deny anyone the pleasure of seeing his dear children go to mass'. If he had been from the same middle-class background as his wife, he may have been able to make a clean break or to adopt a more reasonable attitude to counter the pressures placed upon the family. Moreover, his family might have been in a better position to understand what it meant for them to be a mixed-religion couple and might then have allowed this daughter-in-law to have some say in the matter.

Even in couples where the partners are of the same social standing, however, specific differences to do with the cultural and religious aspects of their relationship can arise, particularly in conflicts which, if they are allowed to go on unchecked, can lead to their breaking up. Is it not the case that when the partners give little thought to any religious convictions, their marriage has more reasons, objectively speaking, for lasting? It might be thought that the absence of religious observance on the part of both partners would guarantee the permanence of their relationship. But there is always the social group to remind them regularly and in a profound way of this religious identity. As Germaine Tillion says, 'the religious factor is dominant. (. . .) Religious barriers are far more solid than national barriers even if one of the partners is not a believer, because religion has a way of affecting things even where there is no religious belief'.[4] Indeed religion does not only have to do with active observances; it is also seen in attitudes, expressions and in the somewhat cryptic way people adopt positions on various matters.

Apart from religion, the status of women can be at the heart of what are sometimes very painful marital problems for some couples. For example, in a Franco-N.W. African couple living in France, the Muslim husband may, to an extent, allow certain attitudes and behaviour in his French wife. He may sometimes be irritated by these, but will nevertheless put up with them until the day when he finally explodes, saying something he had never have dared say before because it would invite disapproval from the majority social group:

> Okay, so I'm not a good dancer, but that's no reason for a woman to make an exhibition of herself all evening with a stranger. She's really gone too far. The way he took her by the arm was somewhat exaggerated. I would go so far as to say impudent. My wife would say that I'm just jealous! (N.W. African, aged 35).

This man feels hurt by the situation described above and interprets it as a conscious effort on his wife's part to create a distance between them. He also resents her behaviour which he sees as a public offence. What he says clearly shows a distinction in his mind between male and female roles, a distinction which is far more apparent in some countries and societies. He would never allow his wife to do the same thing in front of his own people. The relationship between husband and wife there is very codified and limited. There is not only the fact that certain types of behaviour are thought to be out of place, particularly when they are performed in front of 'other people', especially if these 'other people' are men, but also the fact that a certain demonstration of affection towards his wife could give the impression of a loss of masculine identity:

> When we're on holiday, amongst his own people, I get the impression that I no longer exist for him (French woman, aged 32).

To an extent, however, situations of this type occur with non-mixed couples when differences having nothing to do with religious affiliation are highlighted.

A doctor in a small town, with a fairly large rural register of patients, had married his housekeeper. After the first two happy years of marriage together and the birth of two children, the couple's relationship gradually deteriorated. The woman whom he had taken 'out of her farm' had made a great effort to adopt a lifestyle which was far removed from that of her original social group. Their financial situation meant that she was able to engage a woman to help in the house, and she took advantage of this to get involved in cultural activities which did not meet with her husband's approval. Conscious of the social gap between them, she started taking external courses at the Faculty of Arts in a town twenty-five miles away. However, her husband became more and more dissatisfied with her absences which, in his opinion, conflicted with the education plans he had for his children. He found fault with her over it. She took this very badly and fell into a deep depression. It seemed that her husband only wanted her to have the status of the traditional wife and mother at home, sufficiently 'versed in social graces so as not to embarrass him at ordinary middle-class receptions'. She was unable to reconcile what she felt her self to be and the new roles her husband was imposing on her. She took an apartment in the town where she had been studying and which became more attractive to her because of its anonymity. At the same time she started a course of psychotherapy.

The same thing occurred in another couple where the husband, who had become the Managing Director of a company he had set up with a few colleagues, could not come to terms with the fact that his wife had changed so much since their first meeting fifteen years earlier. She was then a secretary. After their marriage she became more and more unhappy with her husband's continual absences, leaving her to keep the home running and bring up their two children alone. Being absorbed with his profession, he too was upset by the fact that his wife should be studying for a professional diploma. Things became even worse when she finished her studies and got a regular job. The division of roles between them was completely out of balance. He no longer recognised the woman he had married. She had changed so much that he was unable to come to terms with it. This comparison between a couple's past and present sometimes becomes a barrier or gulf between the partners. They no longer recognise one another. Their ideas may become more and more divergent. In the second of the two cases referred to above, the husband wanted to run his marriage and family in the same way as he ran his business. The sudden independence achieved by his wife was not only a surprise for him, he was simply unable to accept it because it 'wasn't in accordance with their original contract'.

The sociologist, Andree Michel, illustrates all the changes which may

come about in a couple as soon as a wife engages in some outside
professional activity. 'The woman's work is accompanied by a real
restructuring of the decision making process within a couple.'[5] She adds
that the more a woman becomes involved in the world of work, the more
she challenges traditional roles, both in terms of sex and of family
relationships. Differences appear in the varying levels of incompatibility
which can arise. Arrangements and adjustments on one side, and serious
tensions on the other. This question also arises in mixed couples. It is
settled on the basis of the material resources at the couple's disposal and
on the basis of the communication which exists between the partners and
their ability to develop.

> My husband is the commercial manager in a big company (. . .). Last
> year I taught English in X, then I gave it up to get involved in some
> sport and to start up a jogging club in Z (. . .). He works long hours
> (. . .). He helps me, when necessary, with the children, meals and
> other jobs in the home. He has always helped me (French woman,
> aged 36, married to an American, two children).

The socio-professional level of the husband and their comfortable
financial situation enable this couple to take a more objective view of their
relationship so that the inevitable conflicts can be avoided. Moreover, this
American husband's upbringing means that it is 'natural' for him to help
his wife in the home. This is not the case, however, in another couple
where the husband is from Guadeloupe.

> To begin with we lived together; John hardly did anything to help me
> with daily chores. He thought that it was my job, and was even quite
> demanding about it. Since then we have had two children and he's
> now become very supportive (French woman, aged 28).

In this case the husband's willingness to give a hand with domestic
chores has come about after a period of cultural adaptation. The second
couple cannot be compared with the first. The black man from
Guadeloupe has great difficulty in finding a steady job. He has a certificate
in masonry which he obtained at the end of an FPA (Adult Education)
course, but has often been out of work. Whereas the white American
manager brings home a good, regular salary, the worker from Guadeloupe
is often financially dependent on his white wife who is a secretary.

Thus, given all the varying shades of marital situations in which no
two couples are exactly alike, divorce can strike any couple, mixed or
otherwise.

When a stalemate situation arises, the partners in a mixed marriage feel obliged to resort to the legal sanction of divorce. Whereas for the intra-cultural (non-mixed) marriage divorce is an affair affecting only one group, for a mixed couple it affects two groups, particularly with regard to the children.

Children always remain at the centre of the emotional concerns of the partners. Perhaps people divorce at a later stage in mixed couples, because this break is sometimes accompanied by the departure of the foreign partner to his or her own country. When divorce does not occur early on, the partners may choose to wait until the children grow up. Indeed, the children may for years have been experiencing a difficult emotional balance in the family, feeling a sense of conflicting loyalties between the two parents.

The legal aspect of divorce is very complex and depends on the nationality of the foreign partner. Sometimes it may have been pronounced while the couple are staying abroad in accordance with the law of that particular country. This law may be based on legal customs which are in opposition to those of the other partner. In one country, for instance, polygamy may be permitted, whereas in another country it is absolutely forbidden! The rules of international private law often come up against interminable conflicting procedures, as though each country and each court of law is intent on doing everything it can to substantiate its authority over a member of the group who had removed him or herself in marrying someone of a different nationality.

According to a study carried out by A. Jobert[6] in France, the legal obstacles are different, depending on the nationality of the foreign person who is resorting to a legal remedy. The author devotes a number of pages to divorce and separations in mixed marriages. Out of a total of 248 cases for the year 1974, three-quarters were mixed marriages in which the wife was French. Out of this total, 22% were Franco-N.W. African marriages. Comparing this with divorces in couples where both partners were foreigners, the same breakdown of figures was found to apply. N.W. Africans were followed by Italians, Spaniards and Anglo-Saxons (10%). However, only 2% of Franco-Portuguese marriages ended in divorce. In 70% of cases the marriages were celebrated in France. Care of the children was usually awarded to the mother, even when she was the foreign partner. French law was applied in most cases. The judgments sometimes took account of certain legal procedures used in the country of the foreign partner. However, there is always the delicate question of who should look after the children.

Legal decisions relating to the care of the children, when they have to do with foreign parents, above all in mixed marriages (Franco-Algerian in particular), are the cause of serious tensions, the effects of which exceed the framework of the legal decision itself, and become an issue between the two communities whose interests are sometimes in opposition. The outcome of this type of conflict tends to depend more on the balance of forces and of the actual situation as imposed by one of the partners, than on the objective rights to which the respective partners are entitled.[7]

One thing, however, is certain, and that is the fact that the forces are unfairly arranged for the foreign partner. Every objective and subjective aspect will usually favour the partner who is from that country. What are the reasons for divorce in a mixed couple? According to this author, it would seem that the reasons for such break-ups are not clear-cut. They include those of couples in which both partners are foreign: the role of the woman, the authority of the husband, the way in which children are brought up. However, in this application of French law, certain grievances may be ignored which would not be the case in the country of origin of the non-French partner. A. Jobert points out that court judgments adopt the following formula:

> Since the two partners are of different nationalities, it is necessary to apply French law, as the *lex fori* or relevant law for that location, in terms of the fundamental conditions for divorce.[8]

## And the Child?

The child of a mixed couple becomes a point of contention at two levels, being a very strong bond between the parents, but also a link between the two communities. In the event of a divorce, the child may feel caught between the two sides, even being fought over when the parents do not have sufficient intelligence to settle their post-divorce relationship, thus causing the child to suffer the pain of their disagreements.

> I had never envisaged being separated from my two children (French woman, aged 35, divorced).

However, the father, who was British, was also strongly attached to them. They had to come to a difficult arrangement. Moreover, the physical distance between the two ex-partners makes it difficult to exercise the right of access. When the ex-partner lives more than 1,500 miles away, the child needs to travel by plane to see the father when their holidays do not coincide. Often some partners do not wish to be restricted to the role of visitor and 'provider of maintenance'.

Painful cases sometimes appear in the newspapers, portraying the real suffering people have to go through. One example is the seven year old boy returned to his mother after four years.[9] Married to a N.W. African in 1973, this French woman had been awarded the care of her two children when she was pregnant with a third. The partners nevertheless decided that they would make another attempt at living together and went on a trip to Algeria. During the trip, the father realised that he was going to lose his children, and his family was a source of great pride for him. Before returning to France he entrusted his oldest child, the three year old boy, to his brother. The couple were then divorced and the French wife lodged a complaint. Her ex-husband was condemned on three counts, the third of which involved a prison sentence. He served a few months of the sentence before authorising the return of his son who enjoyed Algerian nationality when in Algeria. Prison was the only expedient the French judges had for enabling the mother to get back her son from a father who had acted in accordance with what he thought he was entitled to do before his own group. The child was brought to France by an Algerian consulate official. This case did not take on exaggerated diplomatic proportions. Nevertheless the suffering lasted a number of years and meant a desperate struggle between the two ex-partners. The child was returned in tears to his mother who no longer recognised him after the three years he had lived with his uncle in Algeria.

This case is not of course entirely typical, but it serves well to illustrate how difficult it is to settle an emotional dispute. Moreover, the legal systems can do little to alleviate this, given the actual state of legislation in different countries. This can be seen in the case of a French father who cannot see his son any more. After divorcing his Austrian wife, she returned to live in Vienna with their child. He went on a hunger strike. It is true that Austria had signed the Franco-Austrian legal convention of 8th April 1967, but it could not effectively enforce the decision of the Paris court in the case of a mother who had asked that her husband renounce his right to see their son again.

A French engineer is being sought by Interpol because he has failed to return his daughter who was awarded to the care of her mother before the divorce went through. Another man cries tears of happiness at seeing his daughter again in Canada after three years of separation. He is however being sought by the Canadian courts for child abduction, a crime which can be punished with fifteen years' imprisonment in that country.

Judges who deal with matrimonial matters have cases of 'divorced children' on their files which, if not quite as spectacular as the cases referred to above, nevertheless involve a certain dramatic element. A private detective agency has been set up to 'recover children being kept illegally by foreign partners'. These agents go to various countries literally to 'kidnap' the children back and return them to the parent entrusted with their care. Parents have to pay great sums for this service. At the International Legal Office set up in Place Vendome in 1971, there are hundreds of files on children who are being fought over by parents who, unable to come to an agreement, are leaving it up to their national judges to pass judgment over irreconcilable jurisdictions. There were 75 cases in 1977, 130 in 1978 and 200 in 1979: the numbers are increasing year by year.

We see an ever faster progression of family life towards separation and divorce at different levels, the development of abductions by air and the cutting down on careful controls at national frontiers which allow this kind of activity to increase. At the same time, the legal systems of different countries retain their national idiosyncracies which are sometimes taken to the point of intransigence. This is the case in Denmark where a mother can still refuse a father the right to see his child. There are signs of change, however. The conference on international private law at The Hague will make a study each year of the conventions in effect between member countries. It will also restrict the rights of the kidnapping parent. In West Germany an association of people has set up *SOS Legal Kidnapping* in Cologne; this is a telephone service which provides assistance to parents whose rights have been encroached upon.

In an official capacity, the International Legal Office of the Ministry of Justice is attempting, through bi-lateral agreements, to facilitate the recognition of legal judgments and their enforcement. These have to do with the law relating to the care of children, the right of access, the right to harbour or shelter children, and other rights. Moreover, the big international organisations, the Commission of Human Rights, the Council of Europe and the Conference on International Private Law in The Hague, are conducting intense campaigns in the interest of these children who are the victims of national barriers. In addition, lawyers often act as effective mediators in the settlement of difficult conflicts.

The problem of national borders is a very real one for children from divorced families, because the interests and distance between the former partners are involved. These matters cannot always be settled 'amicably', as might be the case when both partners live in the same town and cooperate in the joint care of their children. In the case of divorce in a mixed marriage extreme solutions are geared towards exclusive care. As with problem-free marriage, divorce which does not involve considerable problems may be a luxury to which few partners in mixed marriages can aspire.

A breakdown in a relationship leading to divorce assumes a higher profile than is the case in a non-mixed marriage, and it can be more dramatic: 'We are getting divorced just when our house is being built' (French woman, aged 32, two children).

This divorce is all the more noticeable because the identity of the social group had been compromised when the couple challenged it at the start of their relationship.

In a non-mixed divorce the breakdown of the relationship can be seen more as a failure on the part of two individuals, and not as a failure of two groups who thereby underline the lack of understanding between themselves. They married for love, thinking themselves to be alone in the world; they divorce in the cruel reality which enables the social groups to highlight the infallibility of their rules and rights. This social infallibility was involved in their individual waywardness. Their divorce again points to the social importance of matters which were hidden by the initial blindness of their attraction to something different. After a period in the wings, the social group now returns to the centre of the stage with great force. It invades what had been perceived as an intimate freedom. The lovers now realise that their freedom also had a social side to it: 'We told you . . . You couldn't really turn your back on us and on the ways our people have lived for decades'. Divorce always strengthens the position of the social group to the detriment of individual initiative.

Thus, making a clean break always has this sting in its tail, unless the partners decide to stay together, living in a stalemate situation, without resorting to a straightforward divorce. If the legislation on divorce is more obvious for mixed marriage, it is not absolutely obligatory for non-mixed marriages where the stalemate may accompany the partners to the end of their lives without their needing to appear before the courts.

Each couple, however, has to come to terms with this breakdown in the relationship. Some marriages continue in a stalemate situation, others slowly deteriorate. Similar mechanisms exist in mixed marriages, though they are often more intense.

Divorce in this type of marriage is subject to the same parameters as those present at the time of its formation. This is why many divorces took place in connection with Franco-American marriages after the First and Second World Wars. Once difficulties have been overcome, on the other hand, the couple may have summoned up enough energy for ensuring a happy future. A study carried out in the state of Iowa (U.S.A.) showed that the success rate for mixed-religion marriages was in some cases higher than that for marriages between people of the same religion. The same study also showed that where partners state that they have no religious affiliation, divorce occurs more frequently. Religious observance, even when the partners do not share the same religion, is a factor in favour of stability in marriage.[10]

In an earlier investigation (1953) carried out in the state of Iowa, the researchers had already come to the provisional conclusion that 'a mixed marriage in which one of the partners was a Catholic was only half as likely to end in divorce as a marriage between two Catholics'.[11] It was possible to carry out these studies in Iowa because it was one of the first to record the religious affiliation in the marriage and divorce documents. Strong religious practice on the part of one of the partners is able to 'sublimate' a couple's relationship and contribute towards a process of mutual adaptation. Again in the same U.S. state, but in a more recent study, covering a period of thirty years, it was established that marriages between blacks and whites were more stable than marriages in which both partners were black, and that the divorce rate is lower than among white couples.[12] These studies are too sketchy (and in some cases, too out of date) for us to be able to extrapolate anything for the divorce rates in other countries where it is difficult to obtain the necessary statistics.

In terms of the mixed couple itself, it is precisely because it is so difficult for them to settle certain conflicts that such marriages end in divorce. Their attitude in the face of the crises of life is not always negative, however. 'Forewarned' of what is likely to come between them, the partners may be more on their guard when the romantic glow of their first encounter has worn off. They are aware that they got married 'against all evidence'. Because they are a mixed couple, they may perhaps be more likely to tackle crises and disagreements with a less passionate approach.

I would say that when any disagreement occurs in a marriage, the sort of disagreement which can crop up in any type of marriage, it will be aggravated by the fact that the partners have different origins. One might also say that when there is agreement, it is deepened and enlarged when the two partners are not of the same origin, because at that point they are able to experience a kind of alliance against a hostile world, and this has the effect of uniting and consolidating their marriage.'[13]

Taking control of crises, and dealing positively with conflicts and disagreements are tasks every mixed couple has to face up to, as we shall see in the next chapter. This building process is part of the normal dialectic game whose goal is the acquisition of a certain level of maturity in marriage which is needed by all couples. The dynamics of such a relationship make demands on the partners. Though they are certainly characteristics of a mixed marriage, they are just as relevant to the partners of a non-mixed marriage!

**Notes to Chapter 12**

1. *Gros Câlin* [The Big Wheedler]. Paris: Mercure de France, 1974.
2. In his book *Le Mariage dans la Société Française* [Marriage in French Society]. Paris: PUF, 1975, p. 367.
3. Source: INED, 'La conjoncture démographique', [The demographic conjuncture], *Population*, July 1983, No. 4–5. One can also read about divorce in the work by J. Commaille, *Le Divorce en France* [Divorce in France] (with respect to the 1975 reforms and the sociology of divorce). Documentary Notes and Studies, No. 4478, La Documentation Française [French Documents], 1978, as well as the study by Catherine Rager, *Le Temps du Divorce* [Time for Divorce], Paris: Casterman (EPE), 1982, 167 pp.
4. Interview with A. Barbara, in the *France-Culture* broadcast: *'Que sait-on des mariages interraciaux?'* [What do we know about interracial marriages?], 14th January 1977.
5. *Activité Professionnelle de la Femme et Vie Conjugale* [Women's Professional Activities and Married Life]. Paris: CNRS Editions, 1974, p. 64.
6. *Les Étrangers et la Justice Civile* [Foreigners and Civil Justice]. Paris: Credoc, 1976, 213 pp.
7. The same work, p. 59.
8. The same work, p. 51.
9. Case reported by *Ouest-France*, 6th December 1977.
10. Source: L.G. Burchinal and L.E. Chancellor, 'Survival rates among religiously homogamous and interreligious marriages'. *Social Forces*, May 1963.
11. J.P. Monahan, 'Are interracial marriages really less stable?'. *Social Forces*, XLVIII/4, 1970, pp. 461–473.
12. L.E. Chancellor and J.P. Monahan, 'Religious preferences and interreligious mixtures in marriages and divorces in Iowa'. *American Journal of Sociology*, LXI, 1955, pp. 233–239.
13. G. Tillion, ibid.

# 13 Crisis and dialogue

*'I can't stand you any more'*

A mixed couple will be unprepared for crisis and for achieving the desired level of quality in their relationship. Because of its special and sometimes exaggerated nature, crises in such marriages differ from crises in non-mixed marriages. There is a danger that the partners will argue along completely divergent lines. The only possible meeting ground often becomes the venue for short-circuits in communication. Relationships at such times can be somewhat delicate, as well as being destructive for both partners. It is here that the psychology of the foreign partner — the one who lives in the other partner's country — is brought out into the open with all its idiosyncracies. The foreigner is placed in a minority situation, opposite a partner who, although also being a single individual, nevertheless belongs to the majority group.

Through these two individuals it is actually two groups which are engaged in argument, and one side has an unfair advantage. These conflicts often involve strategies, conscious or unconscious, which reveal the respective social and cultural status of each party. Which partner is the dominant one in the relationship? The minority partner will often appear as being in the wrong, knowing that the other partner will always have the social group as a last resort.

Some situations will go as far as destroying the other partner. Intolerable or unacceptable proposals may be put forward, revealing what is nothing less than marital racism, and this may take the form of the hostile relationship between the two groups to which the partners belong. The term 'polack' used by a wife in a heated quarrel is an unbearable insult to her Polish working class husband who has lived in France for the last thirty-five years. She is referring back to an historic balance of forces in which the Pole was not only a poor immigrant, in financial terms, but also an inferior person with a debased alien status. 'To drink like a polack' brings back a past which has unpleasant connotations. It was the image of the drunkard that people associated with the Poles in those days, rather than that of Jean-Paul II or Lech Walesa! This verbal attack recreates, within the couple itself, a situation of destructive mistrust which was experienced both socially and historically in the confrontation of these majority and minority groups: the poor Poles, fleeing poverty, and the French, in need of cheap labour.

'You're all the same!' This expression may trivialise the identity of the other person if it takes the form of a sudden outburst. The other person is suddenly 'aligned' with the identity — usually derogatory — of a group whose status of social equality may have taken decades to achieve. The destructive consequence of this is that anything one may have attributed to the other group in a positive sense is knocked down or undone in a moment.

When the partners in a non-mixed couple resort to such expressions as 'you're mad, I can't stand you, etc.' it is possible for them to interpret the other's meaning because they share the same language. They are able to make allowances by under-valuing the intrinsic meaning of the words used. They are able to place them in a context where they have a different meaning.

In a mixed couple, on the other hand, the levels of decoding become blurred and can even produce 'short-circuits'. The language of anger may be taken at face value by the partner for whom this is not their mother tongue. They will often require time to place these expressions in their right context, at the decoding level intended by the partner. In the same way, a French woman whose husband calls her a 'bitch' may be shocked if she does not correctly interpret this term in her British husband's linguistic framework.

This act of mental juggling with language does not, of course, always take place instantly and it sometimes requires explanations. Misunderstandings occur in verbal and, sometimes, physical attacks and quarrels; they then multiply and increase the chances of creating further misunderstandings. A dynamic process, sparked off by these differences, may then be set in motion unless one of the partners has a moment of clear thinking. If not, it may become impossible to bridge the gulf that has developed between the partners.

Crisis in a mixed couple is nothing more than a concentrated summary of crisis in all couples. What it succeeds in doing, however, is to highlight things which may lie hidden for a long time in non-mixed couples. Crisis provides a true analysis of a couple: a rapid, momentary — yet accurate

— reflection of the true state of relations between the partner. The violence of the conflict causes masks to slip. Social, personal and stereotyped camouflaging is penetrated . . . allowing us to see the true relationship of the couple, stripped of its respectable veneer and reduced to essentials. The formal, outward aspects concealed and contained what was at the heart of the couple, the fundamental base on which their relationship was built. Moreover, the true personality of the partners surfaces from the unexplored depths. The other person is suddenly revealed in a new light, different from what one had always imagined. The outcome will now depend on whether this 'new light' can be accepted.

A foreigner will not always be able to appreciate the significance of swear-words. For him swear-words are just like other words, so he may use them without realising he is doing anything to cause a reaction in people. The person he is speaking with, on the other hand, may take offence because he places the swear-word in the overall context of his mother tongue, aware of all the connotations its usage has (British man, aged 32).

Is the partner rejected when he is suddenly revealed to be different? 'I'd never imagined he could be like that; I'm even surprised at myself that I could be so wrong about him' (French woman, aged 32).

Will a couple who have been brought up short by their own violence be able to re-establish their relationship as a couple, or will they remain locked up in their initial impressions? It is a question of recognising the other person as they appear today, with their true identity. The negative aspects of this new truth become an obstacle for reconsidering the other person and appreciating them for what they are. It is also necessary for the partners to take into account the dramatic expression of the crisis itself in the context of the mixed nature of the couple, the cultural difference and the foreign partner's status as an exile to a certain extent.

Crisis also acts as a point of focus for a more extensive conflict which two individuals find difficult to tackle alone because of the objective differences which divide them. A number of factors affect each partner in a marital crisis situation. In a mixed couple there are the obvious questions of interpretation and cultural translation. As far as this goes, being mixed increases the problems encountered in analysing and resolving conflicts.

A crisis will go through various stages. To begin with the deep causes are often hidden behind the immediate 'reason' before they come out into the open. Different lifestyle, for instance, may be the real reason for a conflict. The husband may be used to keeping late hours; he may make up for this by taking a nap in the daytime. His wife, on the other hand, may be more inclined to go to bed early. Their different sleep needs result in confrontation, friction and fatigue. A tired body very quickly becomes a battleground for crises. Different views on money are also a frequent cause. The apparent lack of worry on the part of one partner can add to the constant worry of the other partner when it comes to managing the household budget. Depending on the couple's income level, disagreement can arise about the very nature of expenses incurred. What one partner buys as a whim may be interpreted as a waste by the other partner. Even space, in small flats, can become a cause of tension.

> My wife has never understood my need for a minimum amount of space around me in our flat. I now see that this space has a symbolic value for me. I thought of it as a place in which I could be truly at home, to make up for my homeland from which I am exiled. With certain limitations, of course, I was able to feel at home again. But she could not understand this. She was always encroaching on my territory, either to tidy up my papers or to change things round. It's caused one argument after another and I find it very irritating (foreigner, aged 42, married to a French woman).

This man is relating how his space, which is very important to him, has not been respected by his wife. She was unable to gauge the importance he attached to it. To give it up would mean to surrender himself. This type of conflict is also, of course, present in non-mixed couples. Here, however, it is amplified and made more specific by the fact that the couple is a mixed one: in his exile, one of the partners has resorted to making special use of the space within his home. Two cultures are in opposition here with regard to the way one's living space should be used. This man finds it essential for his mental and emotional health to feel at home in his living space.

The division of power, when not fairly balanced, can also give rise to crises. The dominated partner suddenly realises that he or she has been robbed of something and rebels, especially if the powers of the dominant partner are exercised over the children. Indeed an uneven struggle tends to favour the partner who is living in his or her own country. The other partner may then become all the more watchful and jealous of the initiatives and prerogatives which they are not allowed in the management of their joint affairs. Nor should we overlook the crises that can come about as a result of sexual misunderstandings where there are incompatible expectations, firmly entrenched views and lack of communication.

The immediate reason for the conflict gives way automatically to the crisis itself. The repetitive aspect of the conflict becomes firmly established and shows how impossible it is to get over. The crisis resurfaces because the reasons for it have not been correctly analysed. In one couple, married for more than twenty years, it is always lack of sleep which, having succeeded in annoying the partners and putting them in a bad mood, results in friction. Nevertheless their areas of disagreement are very deep. The husband has been going for psychoanalysis for a number of years. His wife is very suspicious of such practices. The result is a regular repetition of the same crises.

The same causes and reasons always result in the same crises! However, the way the conflict develops will be subject to endless variations depending on the partners who will make something dramatic, childish or simply ridiculous of it unless they are checked. However, pain and suffering feed on times like these! The level of maturity of the partners will prolong or shorten the period of tension. What we are dealing with here is the way in which people handle conflict. Whether consciously or unconsciously, it will contain the same elements: the opening and closing rites, the ceremony, the stereotyped phrases, the strategy characterising the escalation of verbal or physical violence, the taking and surrendering of ground between the partners, and the lulls. This process of handling conflict may be developed into tactics for resolving what is nothing less than marital warfare. What point is there in continuing to use words when their ambiguity or cruelty have shattered a breakdown situation once and for all? A more physical approach, using tender gestures may serve to remove the barriers or ramparts set up because of a lack of understanding. The language of the body can make up for the insufficiency of words alone. It can back them up and enrich them:

> We didn't speak for ten days following a violent crisis in our relationship. We slept in different rooms. The situation was becoming more and more intransigent; things were actually getting worse because lack of sleep was causing us to lose all sense of balance. The children were witnesses to our ridiculous quarrels. We were behaving like stubborn adolescents. Neither of us wanted to give in. One morning in the bathroom he helped me to do up my bra, something he'd never done before! That was it. I fell into his arms crying. That lunch time we started to talk and our defences began to drop. That evening we made love with real enjoyment. Only in the days that followed did we get round to discussing, in an unheated way, the deep-rooted reasons for our crisis in an attempt to improve our relationship. It is also a fact that if I had not allowed him to do up

my bra, the crisis would have gone on as before (French woman, aged 45, married to a foreigner).

This woman told me that from that day on her attitude to her husband changed. She no longer refused his sexual advances when she didn't 'feel like it'. She accepted the idea that they could make love before their differences of opinion had been explained and clarified. To refuse him and sleep in a different room would be like a 'punishment or retaliation' inflicted on him, and that would have been unbearable.

Once the partners had gained sufficient clarity of thought and were able to stand back a little from their situation, the crisis became a precious moment for restructuring their relationship: they could then look for other ways to relate to one another. This experience gained from learning to handle crises gives some couples the wisdom and serenity which prevent them from taking decisions at the most critical stage of the conflict. A violent crisis, at its most critical stage, is by nature a break in continuity, a disruption.[1] When each partner adopts a strategic position, this only results in mistakes, tensions and hardened attitudes. This then involves holding on to one's personal advantage in a fiercely fought battle between opposing forces. This momentary situation of two-fold disturbances removes all trust and reliability from the decisions taken. On the contrary, the decisions taken in this frame of mind aggravate the crisis, create further obstacles and even result in a stalemate situation.

Deeply angered by her husband's refusal to sleep in the same bed as her, one woman took it upon herself to fold up the camp bed he had set up in his office. She did not see him again for a month. The partners were ensnared by their own decisions: they were their own victims and would almost inevitably have to face the consequences. 'If only I'd known', said the woman. If the partners in this particular case could have stood back a little from their situation, it would have enabled them to appreciate the true significance of their dispute, instead of allowing themselves to be dominated by it. A marital sickness requires that one place the symptom of the crisis to one side in order that one might come up with solutions which do more than aggravate the situation or create a stalemate!

In restructuring their marriage, the partners will be able to analyse their relationship. Is it one of total dependence, to the advantage of the privileged partner in terms of religion, nationality or due to the fact of living in one's own country? Not wanting to relinquish monopoly in terms of power, that partner may attempt to convince the other 'that it is better this way' because it simplifies things. Is it a relationship of independence? It may involve the balance of powers in which the partners arrange their life together and the life of their children on the basis of opposing powers. Often the resolution of their hostile conflicts takes the form of a war of attrition. Prisoners to the principle of not giving in, the partners become more and more distant and indifferent to one another. Independence has led them to indifference. A relationship of interdependence can become one which gives birth to neutrality, and non-involvement between them. They then come to arrangements on the division of powers. The conflicts are settled as though they were contracts. Aware of their separation, the partners look for crossroads at which they can meet for certain moments of intense exchange, as though these were emotional parentheses in their lives. Their love relationship is more in evidence at moments of understanding than in the ongoing heaviness of their lives together.

For partners in mixed marriages, however, where each has his or her own characteristic differences, the needs are greater than in non-mixed couples. A good relationship, which is deeply sensitive to the real identity of each person, is able to bring both partners together in unity. This type of relationship establishes a channel of communication between the partners. Power is shared, and conflicts are more like warnings than fully fledged accusations. The crisis is just one factor among a number of others. It is, of course, difficult but it is only an expression of confrontation in the context of changes taking place within the couple. The partners will endeavour to come through the crisis, rather than allow themselves to remain stuck there indefinitely.

This distinctive type of relationship brings together two individuals who wish to understand one another's differences, without losing out in terms of the spontaneous, cultural expression of their feelings for one another. Just as this type of relationship makes it possible to handle crises effectively, it also enables the couple to manage their own relationship overall. Being aware of their objective differences and of their different points of view on a number of matters, the partners devote time and thought to their marriage relationship, allowing plenty of scope for improvisation. Improvisation is possible because space is made for it. It is grafted onto an already structured relationship within the couple on the basis of parameters which both partners have clearly defined and made their own.

This marital 'distinctiveness' is of course necessary in a mixed marriage because it quite clearly refers to two individuals who are foreigners to one another; but it is just as applicable to non-mixed couples in that it enables them to move from a state of inert conjugality (in which the partners are permanently fixed) to a state of open conjugality, making it possible for them to develop together in harmony with their respective interdependent developments. But how does one achieve this 'distinctiveness' in a relationship?

It is the result of a certain skill in a couple's married life. We have already seen, with reference to the mixed couple, how communication requires an apprenticeship in communication skills and in the art of interpretation when one partner does not have the same command of the language of communication. A wish on the part of two individuals to have a deep lasting emotional relationship is not enough in itself. This wish is itself emotional and is therefore subject to change — with peaks and troughs — whereas a skill can be a structure around which feelings can grow. These feelings will be in a far better position to thrive if the partners have looked for the strongest possible support for their expression. Communication skills enable the foreign partners to make the appropriate mental translations when they are speaking. They have become aware, on the basis of analysis, of each other's language structures, levels of meaning, and the way in which their minds and emotions interrelate. Conscious also of the enormous scope for misunderstanding in conversation, they will then be in a position to learn methods and take opportunities to engage in a sort of mutual decipherment (in the same way as twins are able to understand half-spoken thoughts and half-smiles) until an almost complete, unambiguous exchange takes place. They will have available to them a series of intimate relationship skills, and will even perhaps be able to go back to times when their relationship was truly one between fiancés.[2] All these elements, placed side by side in the form of a mosaic, will make up these communication skills, this capacity for living together in a healthy, growing relationship from which humour is not lacking!

Neither of us is actually firmly entrenched in the views of our respective countries, so we are able to see the funny side of the differences between our two cultures. We make fun of the fact that I am 'Latin' and he is 'Anglo-Saxon', in that I am expansive and he is reserved (French school teacher, aged 37, married to an American, aged 38).

The partners will thus create a relationship of freedom based on trust. It will not depend on the dictates of society alone for its survival. Does this mean that the partners will devote all their energy to combating the fundamental areas of opposition in order to establish their self-contained identities? Being neither complementary nor opposed to one another, each partner will be recognised for his or her *significant difference* and the way in which that is expressed. These differences are not accepted just as they are, but because they are understood and reinterpreted, without prejudice, in terms of the other partner's cultural system. Instead of separating them, the partners try to find a carefully assessed way of articulating these differences. Thus, this distinctive relationship does not shut up the other person in a determinist category. On the contrary, it enables the two partners to distinguish between culture and nature. The other person is not accepted at face value; instead they are recognised and understood for themself, as a person, within their deep, cultural frame of reference. They are recognised and truly understood in a face-to-face encounter. This relationship makes it possible to pass from one level to another, from zero level in their marriage to a marital existence of quality. It *confers identity*[3] on each partner. In their face-to-face encounter they are both built up and strengthened as people. Moreover, because of their intimate marriage relationship, a *marital identity* is also conferred on them.

But where does desire come into all this? Desire certainly exists. It is channelled, however immersed, in the social context. The partners live out their various daily relationship (financial, emotional, sexual) and their desires within a social context. Their intimate world is of course built up in a unique way, yet in this they are like other couples. Indeed their emotional relationship will take shape around the ever-increasing recognition of the differences they discover, differences which transcend their way of giving and receiving so that they can be fully themselves.

The foundations for this type of relationship will be based on a dynamic bond which is in a state of continual renewal. There will then be times, in certain areas, when the partners will be able to say, without deceiving themselves: 'We are alike; we are not so different — we have the same desire'.

It is not so much the objective or intrinsic difference which introduces a sense of distance between people; rather it is one's point of view on the matter. Once recognised for what it is, difference is no longer a reason for areas of divergence to come about between them.

I now realise that my wife perceives this difference as something belonging to me. And she respects it in me; she is curious about it and asks me what it feels like from my point of view (British man, aged 30, married to a French woman).

What we see here, then, is a relativisation, if not an appreciation of difference, and this can form common ground for encounters between the partners, ground in which they can take root together.

From the start I was interested in things American; I got to know all I could about it and can appreciate American literature in the original (French woman, married to an American).

This 'marital distinctiveness' becomes a true blending of the elements which go to make up the identity and personality of each partner. It gives them the chance to live out their life as a couple, not so much in a marital territory which is separated by the party wall of indifference or marital *apartheid*, that is to say a contract of individual sufferance, but in a space where they are able to recognise and understand one another.

Does this mean that crisis can be avoided? Not exactly. But the relationship is characterised by a control or mastery of the crisis so that it becomes something which is seen at more of an objective distance. The partners gradually learn how to manage it once they have understood from experience how conflicts can begin, develop and end. 'If we're not careful here, it's going to turn into a real crisis' (woman, aged 40). Instead of being damaged, surprised or wounded by it, they will be able to channel their energies, not so much towards avoiding it at all costs, but towards facing up to the situation honestly. They will then be in a position to relativise the conflict and see it more in perspective: by analysing the different factors involved and the relative positions of each partner in the heat of the moment when the situation is at its most painful.

This ability to stand back somewhat from the situation comes from training in the management of one's own marital conflicts, taking into account the intensity of the moment and the length of time over which a situation has developed, just as an individual — instead of staying on a collision course with serious ill health — will manage his body and continually monitor his symptoms and indications of improvement. This calm confrontation of crises is a critical process and it saves people from falling into the usual stereotypes of conflict. These stereotypes are repeated because the partners have not made a conscious effort to avoid them. To break this repetitive cycle and the inevitable wear on the marriage, by standing back and taking a more objective view of things, makes of the crisis an area in which a solution can be found on the basis of certain conditions, at the appropriate time, and in a way which will not allow the situation to worsen.

It is only natural that if one partner places the other at a distance, the level of frustration, pain and, thus, aggression will increase. Once a certain period of time, needed by both partners, has elapsed, one of them will have to take the initiative to resolve the situation. In this sense, the crisis is a return to adolescence. But when they succeed in dismantling these mechanisms of behaviour, the partners will no longer be the objects of their own crises; they will instead be the subjects. Then they will be able to prevent crises from attacking them.

What we are describing is a new type of attitude, an adult way of behaving in the context of an event which is quite often characterised by aggressive reactions. This new attitude is what distinguishes the 'distinctive' relationship which allows each partner his or her own autonomous space, while keeping a control on possible areas of friction and attack.

This 'distinctiveness' is a carefully thought out approach in a marriage at two different levels: it is a conscious attitude on the part of the couple as well as on the part of each partner. Moreover, it is the basic element for the couple's coming to terms with their social context as they work out, in time and space, the duality of their relationship in terms of their emotional and sexual natures.

This relationship can bring about a new way of looking at the other person. The individual/object now becomes a person, a subject/being living alongside the other person, both for him or herself and for that other person, in a fully reciprocal process. One partner therefore becomes 'someone' — a unique individual — for the other partner. There is no longer any place for one person living in another's shadow. This new type of attitude is both a dynamic support and a commitment in which the needs resulting from a person's desires are to be met: 'Every day I ask myself how I am dealing with my own desires and with his' (woman, aged 45).

**Notes to Chapter 13**

1. E. Durkheim uses the term *anomy*, particularly in his study on suicide.
2. From the old French word *fiancé*, meaning 'the state of a soul which has trust'.
3. Expression borrowed from Mr de Certeau.

# 14 Cultural mix and social mix

*'She is the closest of distant women'*

Where does the fact of being a mixed couple come into all of this? Why concentrate so much on mixed couples or marriages when, as we have seen, the qualtiy of a dual relationship does not differ significantly between a mixed couple and a non-mixed couple? 'Mixed marriage' is in itself a dangerous term, because it enshrines an idea, or an ideology. It would be far more appropriate to use the term *intercultural* marriage to describe this type of marriage which brings two foreign individuals together. It is actually more significant to speak of cultural mix with respect to this type of marriage.

Mixed marriage is at the centre of the relationship between the individual and his social group of origin. Should it be regarded as deviant when most marriages are concluded within the group? Why marry outside of the group? Is it the 'loosening of social ties' as the sociologist Durkheim puts it, which brings about such marriages with foreigners? Should people be regarded as *anomic* for contravening the social standards of the group and showing a certain amount of distance, if not breaking away? But a mixed marriage is the consolidation of a distance which already existed between an individual and his or her group. A French woman, depending on her position in the social hierarchy, may look at her marriage to a foreigner differently and place great importance on her relationship of love. The fact of having left her country for a foreigner who has come to Europe or France, is not a neutral one: it is the result of a strategy aimed at finding employment, or a result of forced or chosen emigration, as is the case with certain students from the Third World. For such a foreigner, marriage to a French woman represents an additional factor in adaptation and assimilation, alongside his work or studies. By marrying a French woman, he is at the same time marrying France.

From the standpoint of the social group, the rights of the couple may be recognised in terms of their love for one another, but at the same time they may be censured in social terms.

However, the creation of mixed marriages also obeys certain social rules which they have in common with non-mixed marriages. For example, in France the large proportion of marriages with Italians, Spaniards and N.W. Africans at times when immigration levels have been high explains the link between such marriages at certain times and not at others. In the same way there were many Franco-German marriages at the end of the War. The migrations involved when people go on holiday and when military operations are being carried out can also favour such marriages. According to the studies conducted by A. Girard and L. Roussel, half the marriages taking place in France are between partners of the same or very similar social background. Mixed marriages do not escape these rules. The son of a foreign ambassador is not at all likely to marry the daughter of an ordinary French worker.

Let us take as an example the case of a young girl from a family of doctors: employed as a secretary, because she had failed to get a degree, she had ambitions, not to marry a man in a similar position to herself, but to marry a doctor who would regain for her the social status she felt she was beginning to lose. If she were to marry a black African doctor, she would again rise in the social hierarchy, but not so quickly and not to so high a level as she would if married to a white French doctor. But in the absence of French doctor, she would stand to gain more from marrying a black doctor than a white male nurse who would rise more slowly and to a far lower level in the social structure.

This example, which is a fictitious one, expresses something of the complexity of two individuals' positions when they decide to become a couple. It focuses attention on the combination of two major areas of mixedness: that of the cultural mix (in which one may encounter all those differences having their origin in nationality, religion and language) and that of the *social mix* (which is essentially the difference in class or social background).

Thus, mixedness is not an entity in its own right; rather it is made up of a wide range of important, independent differences between the partners. However, the objective identification of these differences is not in itself a sign of mixedness. It is the lack of agreement on those differences between the partners which starts to create a gulf between them. This type of difference, therefore, creates distance. In the case of a couple which is mixed socially (heterosocial) living in France, the husband being a shopkeeper and the wife a working woman, the two partners may belong to two different groups, but they will in general have common points of reference, relating to French culture, even if different levels of cultural practices separate them at some points. In a couple which is culturally mixed, on the other hand, there will sometimes be a total mistrust of the social reference groups in each culture. There is the danger that the couple's problems will be dealt with unfairly depending on the social class. There will be a certain social relativism; mastery of the situation will be more difficult for working class couples.

Just like all other marriages, a mixed marriage reveals a number of things about the institution of marriage. Moreover, mixed couples will react to situations in a certain way because they want to 'be like everyone else', not wanting to stand out too much from other couples of the same social background. However, between the strong desire to become assimilated — in effect to deny the difference of at least one of the partners (and the children) — and the reality of the situation, we can identify, among other things, certain cultural elements which are more relevant to mixed marriage than to marriage in general.

When a N.W. African marries a French woman in France, they will be faced with more or less the same problems as those faced by any couple, i.e. integration into a social context which will enable the partners to live together, probably to have children, and not to get divorced. In a Franco-N.W. African couple, the fact of not having regular employment, together with uncertainty about tomorrow, may well be a more significant reason for the couple's breaking up than the fact that they are mixed. A Franco-N.W. African couple from the upper classes (e.g. a doctor and a nurse) will have resources and means for overcoming their difficulties which are not available to a working class couple.

Can the material difficulties of existence be blamed on nationality or on the colour of one partner's skin? Of course the mixed nature of the relationship plays a part and, depending on the social backgrounds, conflicts can be heightened by the importance of the religious culture of the partners, such that the differences of culture and religion can be held up after the event as the reason for given difficulties. They suddenly assume an importance which they had not hitherto enjoyed. The appearance or reappearance of a certain personality type — modelled on the different cultures — is then put forward as the reason for the couple's failure; it is the sort of evidence one is all too ready to take hold of and behind which one can safely shelter. Social difficulties take advantage of the differences between the partners and enforce a sudden pattern on them. Thus the process of disenchantment begins . . . Is this just because the couple is mixed?

We might well consider the very nature of such mixed or *intercultural* marriages. It is of course a marriage like any other, but it brings out a great many more questions. *It is an ordinary, specific marriage.* Its specific nature, however, is significant because the individuals involved, whether they like it or not, bring with them their group of origin, even if at certain points they feel they have severed all links with it. How many marriages which one thought to be well balanced and united become complex when they move abroad. At home, the fact that the couple was mixed was less apparent, they could often go unnoticed, even though problems existed. As soon as one changes the place of residence, various phenomena come to light: the reappearance of the structural link with the group of origin, the return to one's social identity, the reawakening of old allegiances which had been dropped in order to live as a 'loving twosome' or to isolate oneself, as though the couple were passing from its dual phase to its social phase.

If the partners first met in the home country they will have found a whole system of dual and social adjustments to the majority group (that of one of the partners) right from the start of their married life. At its birth, the couple is ready to find a means of integration which satisfies its internal relationship which has assumed a greater priority than the groups surrounding it: 'Alone in the world, with eyes for no one but each other'. This is the period of discovery, romanticism and encounter: the partners forget all about the social reality around them. Moving to another country, to another social group can only be achieved with a certain destructuring of this primary relationship which has come into being since the encounter. Changing from one majority group to another will be difficult for the partner who now finds him or herself alone, and the demands will be greater at the very time when this transplanting of the couple is most threatened by the sudden criticism of the life this couple is leading. A certain wear and tear is added to the erosion of the initial romanticism. The social relationship with the groups in question will take the place (by way of compensation) of a dual relationship which is now weakened, less intense and less solid. The development of this relationship and the distance which creeps in are well expressed in these lines taken from a letter addressed to the magazine *Droit et Liberté* [Law and Liberty]:[1]

> In 1976 I left my country [Mauritania] with the aim of continuing my studies at a university in France, and I duly enrolled for a course. In 1978 I got to know a French girl who was also a student. We fell in

love and the girl decided one day that she would introduce me to her parents. They were very much against the meeting. Her father even went so far as to say that to invite a black man to his home was out of the question. Then came the day when this young woman decided she would marry me and come back with me to Africa; we got married and had a child.

After the birth of our child, my wife's racist family began to interfere in our marriage. They wanted to reproach their daughter for what she had done, and used our son as an instrument in this. My wife has now gone over to her parents' side. She wants a divorce. I am prepared to divorce her, but it will mean losing contact with my son.

The main aim of my wife's parents is to show that mixed marriage is a foolish idea and that black people are incapable of living with so-called civilised people.

Whilst showing the writer's suffering and bitterness, this letter maps out the journey the couple made together. She is white, and he is black. They are both students and fall in love. They decide to get married despite the opposition of the parents. They go off to build their love nest in Africa where the strength of their relationship is able to overcome the passive resistance of the parents. By breaking away from her parents this white woman 'is also tearing herself away from her own community' in order to embrace another in which she hopes to make a cultural conversion. Everything goes well until the birth of their child. It is this new being who will become the link between the generations.

The couple's move to Africa was no doubt decisive in increasing the renewed resistance of the parents, who were now on the offensive for getting their daughter back to the group to which she belonged. Her return was encouraged by the physical separation from her country and from her own people. 'My wife has now gone over to her parents' side. She wants a divorce'.

We see here the journey made by a couple who tried to take things too fast. The first romantic, binding stage found its expression in a state of mind in which pleasure was isolated: 'We are alone in the world; too bad if our parents don't understand'. The second stage is more focused on the duality of the situation: to build up the relationship between the partners and to make plans for the future. Finally the third stage, pregnancy and the birth of the first child, reinstates the importance of the social aspects of life which had been abandoned. It is of course the family which engages in these *social manoeuvres* through the child. The woman swings back to the social group of her own background. She allows herself to be drawn back into her own group because her cultural conversion to the very different group of her husband had been unsuccessful; and this occurred at the very point when the husband was experiencing confirmation from his own people since he had been rejected by his wife's parents. The Mauritanian husband seems to be prepared for divorce, but he too is tied to a group for whom the child is an important link. The conflict between these two individuals is a picture of the conflict between the two groups. At the end of the letter they are pitted against one another: the 'civilised' white parents and the powerless, 'uncivilised' black parents. Mixed marriage becomes a foolish thing because it tries to bring the two together.

This journey may be encountered in an intracultural marriage, but with less haste, of course — for it may have been four years since the couple first met and two years since their official marriage — and with less intensity. The problems of a mixed marriage are by nature the same as those of an 'ordinary' marriage; they are experienced with a greater intensity, however, and with more significant consequences. The solutions are more dramatic or more dramatised, just because of the higher stakes involved. 'It is difficult to admit that you were wrong when a break-up occurs' (French woman, aged 30, one child).

In this sense, mixed marriage does not need a special theory for defining it as a marriage; rather it allows us to gain a clearer understanding of all marriages. It enables us to identify all those areas of mixedness, distance and difference which can exist in any couple. These distances can be perceived, among other things, in the area of age when one partner is a lot older than the other; in the area of health when one of the partners is handicapped; in the area of social status if there is too obvious a difference between the groups to which they belong; and even in the area of marital status when a widowed or divorced person remarries, with or without children.

The mixed — *intercultural* — couple also contributes a range of religious, ethnic and racial differences which produce *a sort of systematic overall shock*. There is, for instance, the matter of choosing names for children, and choosing a decor which will create harmony between, say, Breton furniture and pottery from Kabylia. The sort of music listened to and the way in which time is used may surprise the other person. These systematic, emotional or unexpressed choices have to be handled in daily life. This explains the difficulties encountered, but it also accounts for the richness which can be present.

This type of couple clearly demonstrates for today's generation the difficulty of living in a lasting relationship as a couple. As such, mixed couples provide an interesting setting for the search for an intense lasting encounter: an encounter which is no longer obvious but one which is built up. To a certain extent, the partners of a mixed marriage have an advantage over non-mixed couples. The very nature of their mixedness means that they come into contact far sooner with areas of conflict. This limited advance warning, this acceleration of the process can enable them to react to and deal once and for all with what would try to separate them, so that they are able to invest in the building up of their relationship. The foundations have been explored early on, whereas in the case of non-mixed couples one may have seen marriages which were 'going well' until the fateful crisis which suddenly destroyed the fragile construction of two people 'who seemed to get on so well together'.

Even when in a non-mixed marriage the partners seem to be so similar for a long time, because of what they have in common, they can still suddenly find themselves strangers to one another. In mixed marriages, on the other hand, the partners are in a better position to become quickly aware of their objective differences because of the situations which highlight them. They will then try, not to become similar, but to draw nearer to one another and find points and areas in which they can truly meet one another. A process of consolidation of areas of likemindedness starts to take shape. The initial work involved in clearing the ground can give the partners a true understanding of foundation on which their relationship as a couple is built; as they become aware of their limitations this will encourage them to adopt a line of conduct inspired by a freely chosen progression, whereas for non-mixed couples the direction their relationship takes may be decided more by events.

We see here two different developments. In the non-mixed marriage the apparent (i.e. subjective) and obvious distinctions between the partners will for a long time hide the actual differences between them which are hidden and unidentified until they suddenly come to light. By this time, however, when the fervour of love may not be so intense, the couple will already be of a certain age and will have gone through a number of experiences, with varying levels of success, which will take them on from one stage to the next. In a mixed marriage the early awareness of the distance which actually separates them will lead the partners to ask themselves some basic questions. The fervour of their love, and the emotional investment they have made, may become a reserve from which they can at once draw strength — because there is still time — in order to find the basis for a new consensus. In this way their relationship takes on a new dynamic aspect. It is for this reason, as we have seen, that divorces in mixed marriages occur earlier than in non-mixed marriages.

Given its difficult context, mixed marriage can provide the partners with more opportunity for choice. We might ask another question here: how can anything so distant be experienced in such a close way?

One husband, speaking of his wife with a certain amount of humour, and paraphrasing a well known advertising slogan for a holiday company, said: 'She's the closest of distant women'.


**Notes to Chapter 14**

1. No. 395, October 1980, MRAP monthly publication (The movement against racism and for friendship between peoples).

# 15 The land of settlement

*'Where is our home?'*

The partners of a mixed couple will find it difficult to avoid the question of where they are to live. Do they envisage settling in the country where they met or, perhaps, where they were married? Have they lived together for some years without facing up to this question which will be more difficult to answer for the foreign partner.

The choice of the actual location of their home as a couple and as a family will often face couples in a dramatic way. If they move to the other partner's country, will this not just serve to reverse the dilemma: departure for one partner, and a return home for the other? Once a move has been made, the couple may still come up against this same basic question again: 'Where are we going to live?'

We haven't solved this problem for good. It's a very important question. My husband would like very much to return to Great Britain. It would be easy for him to get a job there. But what would become of me? And what about our two children; I can't imagine them among English children. They are more French than English. They already have their own friends; it would mean completely uprooting them (French woman, aged 32, two children; married to a British teacher).

This woman clearly highlights the difficulty involved in coming up with a solution which suits both partners. The choice of the place of residence becomes an even more delicate one when the children's education comes into the equation. This choice involves the risk of becoming uprooted, as well as the fear of living a different sort of lifestyle. It would seem, in this example, that it would be far easier for the foreign partner to remain in France since he has got used to it over a number of years, than for his wife to have to get used to a strange new world.

In this particular case, the British partner has to an extent put down roots in this provincial French town. It is no longer foreign to him. His neighbours and colleagues think highly of him. He does not suffer from discrimination in any sense; except, of course, when France is playing football against England, and then he catches a glimpse of a rather unpleasant French nationalism. But this is not the norm. In addition there is nothing to distinguish him physically from a Frenchman. He is not black and does not have North African features! Indeed the primary cost of adapting to life in France has now been paid, and his wife dreads paying a similar cost if they were to change countries. She looks around for every possible reason in support of her position, referring to the Frenchness of their children. She even adds:

> Besides, he is not really quite English now, having lived in France for fifteen years. He too would have some difficulty in adjusting to life in England.

She is not altogether wrong. Having left Britain as a single person, he would now be returning with a family. The return to his native land would involve both an adjustment on his part after a long absence, and the acceptance of his wife and children in a country which is foreign to them. This possible move could only become a reality after long, careful consideration and preparation.

> What my wife says is partly true. There are a number of difficulties. I also have a lot of questions about it, and they are a cause for concern. One fear I have is that the move would unsettle my children (British man, aged 33, married to the French woman above).

This Franco-British couple do not have such a dramatic choice to make. After all, France and Great Britain are more or less neighbouring countries. The closeness of the two countries enables the partners to contemplate the choice with a measure of calmness.

However, when the partners are from very distant countries, geographically and culturally, they have a far bigger decision to make. The gulf may become so much a part of their thinking that they will never contemplate returning to the other partner's country because of the difficulties it would involve.

> My wife would never get used to the African bush. And where would we send the children to school? There's no highschool. The issue has really been settled for a long time. I will stay in France with my black skin. I go back home less and less. What matters most now is my family here (Senegalese man, aged 42, married to a French woman).

The desire on the part of one partner to return to his own land raises the question of the couple's identity and its attachment to a given community and place. The mixed nature of the couple is seen here quite clearly. Until this desire is expressed the couple is able to get on with everyday life and to live like other couples around them.

There are a number of often very original compromise solutions which make it possible to preserve the identity of each member of the family. There is, in particular, the important psychological investment in holidays, which has a considerable financial cost. An Italian man, married in France, returns every year to the Abruzzi village he left twenty-five years ago. He always arranges it so that the day before his return from holiday coincides with the traditional festival which brings him into contact with all his childhood friends who, like him, have emigrated from Italy to other European countries, and North America. His family's frequent holidays in Italy are in harmony with his business activities. This man has kept his Italian nationality.

My children are French, of course. They were born in France. It is easier for them: for their studies and for work. But every year they go to Italy and they speak Italian; they enjoy it (Italian man, aged 45, married to a French woman).

The perfect sense of balance achieved by this man, who is known in his town, is due to the frequency of his trips between France and Italy, and the trips made by his whole family. He maintains permanent contact with Italy by telephone or through the numerous visits of his brothers, sisters and cousins who never hesitate to drop in a few days every year. He does not lead an exile existence as is the case for a working man originally from the Aures region in Algeria, who has also lived in France for twenty-five years but has not been back to his poor village at the edge of the Rhoufi[1] for fifteen years.

As far as I'm concerned, it's all in the past. This is now my country, where my children live. I'm also waiting to be naturalised (Algerian man working in the car industry, aged 43, married to a French woman, three children).

This final severing of his roots causes this man to adopt a cultural alignment which is largely determined by his social origins as a peasant and by his present status. He will not of course have a very large holiday budget. He maintains the odd contact with Algerians of his age who also settled in France for financial reasons. Some of them, married to French women, are afraid of the fluctuating laws on immigration which threaten to force them to leave the country. The situation is altogether different for an American director who has lived in France for five years and is married to a French woman. This couple has just had a second child, named Samy.

When we go back to the States, Samy will have no problem being American (American man, aged 33, married to a French woman).

This couple has a relatively easy life. The husband is a commercial director and the multinational company which employs him enables him to make a number of trips a year to the States. His wife speaks American English fluently (and the children hear both languages spoken every day). Her husband's position will make it easier for her when they finally settle in an American city. Interested in American literature and museums, she is already looking forward to her life on the other side of the Atlantic.

The place of residence is often chosen on the basis of where the couple first met and spent their first years together. An attempt at living in the country of the foreign partner may have been made, followed by a return to the first country until the point when, for family, financial or political reasons, the couple finally settles down and begins to invest in a specific location: buying a house, buying heavy furniture, etc. They will make up for this final decision by regular trips and holidays in the other country. Some couples, for whom the experience of living in either of the two countries involved has not been a positive one, may consider settling in a third country. Placed on an equal footing by this choice, the partners will then have a different situation to face. However, such rare cases only occur with adventurous individuals in certain countries where the regulations on immigration are not so strict. It is a question of not creating more difficulties than they would have had if they had stayed in the country of one of the partners.

Settling in whatever country will cause various problems. For instance, the roles of men and women are not seen in the same way in western and eastern countries. The concept of what it means to be a couple may be touched at its most intimate point. Political troubles may suddenly increase the anxiety of the foreign partner and his children. The fear of expulsion will also be a concern. Rejection by the native population is often very marked, particularly in certain countries where foreign women are seen as competitors when students, returning from Europe, come back to their own countries in Africa with a degree and a French wife. The arguments expressed in some press articles in these countries reveal the sometimes precarious psychological situation of these couples.

I didn't have a job in England and my wife had broken off her studies when we got married. It was better for us to return to France. Besides, I had fewer family ties than she did (British man, aged 35, married to a French woman, two children).

This man is a good example of how decisive the financial aspects can be in a couple's lifestyle. It is often the country which offers the better standard of living which the couple will choose. A certain financial ease will facilitate professional and cultural activities, in addition to encouraging good relationships. The couple will be attracted by the group which offers a greater number of family bonds for one of the partners, whilst safeguarding their independence.

So far things have been on a temporary basis. We had had enough of living in a council house. We have now had a house built. I hope to go back to live in England again one day, though. My wife accepts this: after all, I've accepted living here for a number of years. It's only natural that there should be some give and take (*Idem*).

This man feels he has made something of a sacrifice by living in France for a number of years and thinks that his wife is able to make the same sacrifice. But there is no real systematic equation between the first year of married life and those which follow when the problems become more complex because of the children. This sacrifice is likely to be disproportionate for the wife if it is required of her too late in the marriage:

I wouldn't wait too long before deciding to leave France. I would have to do it before it was too late (French woman, wife of the man above).

Mixed couples have very different situations to face depending on their social context. Even if they are from very distant countries, a husband and wife in top managerial positions will be able to enjoy a lifestyle which smoothes over the extreme situations caused by the fact that they are of mixed nationalities. A mixed working class family, on the other hand, will not have the same mobility, due to the lack of financial resources. Certain situations will be very difficult for them. A mixed couple's ability to travel will depend on their income.

This is no problem for us. Our life straddles the border. My husband's business activities in Switzerland do not in any sense make my life as a German woman difficult. We very often visit our second home over the border several times a month. Our children are at home in both countries (German woman, married to a Swiss company director).

But even given the same social context, the great distance often becomes a very difficult obstacle to get over:

> It's not just around the corner, of course. One trip a year with three children is quite expensive enough. There is a considerable imbalance because the children do not see my husband's parents very often (French woman, married to a manager from Guadeloupe).[2]

Settling down in one of the partner's countries involves considerable additional expenses: travel, postage, etc.

> We have already spent 800 Francs in telephone charges this month. It was the Christmas season and Granny and the children wanted to speak to one another on the phone. It is difficult to avoid this (British woman, aged 35).

Such mixed practices will not stop the foreign partner from wanting to return to his own country at some point in the future. The couple will then have to think very objectively about the choice made. A frequent solution to this is for the couple to settle in the country where the family and social constraints are not so strong. The great attraction of the nuclear family encourages the couple to settle where one of the partners is less likely to feel exiled the more he invests, by way of compensation, in the life of his family and children. The less of a foreigner he feels in his partner's country, the more he will be able to accept living far away from his native land.

These questions will last on into old age, extending to the place in which the couple intends to retire:

> I'm old now. It would uproot me completely to live down there. I would lose all my friends. How could you expect me to establish a new circle of friends at my age? (French woman, aged 55, married to an Algerian, living in France for twenty-five years).

This woman is afraid of uprooting herself at this stage in life. Her married children and grandchildren are an additional factor against her leaving France. Her husband thinks differently, however.

> How can you say you won't come with me to spend our retirement in Algeria, when I've devoted more than two-thirds of my life to you? (Algerian, aged 66, married to the woman above).

Some people living in exile come to painful conclusions at the end of difficult journeys through life: for instance, when a N.W. African no longer sees his children after a certain age because they have become fully

French and completely at home with going to mass. He now faces old age alone. He may feel that he has reached a stalemate situation. Without becoming officially divorced he may separate from his wife if she is not willing to go with him to his own country:

> What do you expect? When one grows old, one is gripped by this irresistible urge to go home. I find it unthinkable that I should be buried anywhere other than my village in Kabylia. So, you see, it's something far deeper than reintegration (Algerian from Kabylia, aged 46, teacher).

For this man from Kabylia, the earth of one's native land is important and, as Mouland Feraoun writes, he will hear its 'imperious call' in his old age. It is because he has worked all his life on foreign soil that he will want to return to his own land and find his final resting place there: 'One small grave mixed up with all the others, for it will bear no inscription, and as soon as the first spring comes it will be covered with frail graminaceae and white daisies'.

The choice of where to make one's home involves symbolic representations one cannot imagine and cultural beliefs in a society where the sense of community survives death itself. It is quite certain that this choice has consequences as far as this last resting place for the body. The problem will be less intense in cultures where incineration is the normal practice. The relationship of the individual with his group is measured culturally on the basis of precise indicators among which is the place where the person is buried.

It would seem, therefore, that right until the end the partners in a mixed marriage experience a sort of separation. After having attempted to establish their financial, professional and emotional home, and the home of each of the children, the issue of a retirement home will raise this final question: 'But where are your roots?'

Sadly, the partners sometimes live in a series of disconnected homes. Whatever the location of the home, each partner will have different ways of expressing the concept 'our home' which reveal the irreducible distance between them, even when one partner has opted for the other's camp. That partner will still sometimes find himself thinking in terms of 'them'.

Has either partner made a true rational commitment to 'becoming French, N.W. African or American? In the deep recesses of the mind there will remain pockets of the original hidden identity. What significance does 'our family home' have when the children leave to set up their own homes? Will their homes be based on fragments of transhumance between the need to settle down somewhere out of choice and the choice to settle down out of necessity in the best place to live?

One only needs to run the sequence through a little before coming to the final choice of the best place to die . . . and be buried:

My father was cremated and, since I am an atheist, I'm not at all concerned about where I will one day be buried (British man).

This man lived in an international family environment which may explain his relative disassociation from his roots:

I never really knew a home. My past was quite different from that of my friends. I do not really have any roots (British man).

But will this also be the case for his children who, against the backdrop of the course of life followed by their parents, are forming their own 'childhood home'?

**Notes to Chapter 15**

1.  A canyon in the Aures — a very poor, mountainous area of Algeria.
2.  Although legally French, a person from Guadeloupe is a foreigner from the cultural point of view. See the chapter on different types of mixedness.

# 16 Conclusions

## A Social Existence in a Mixed Condition

By their very existence in society, mixed marriages confront society with the problem of their identity; indeed it is not just the odd marriage of this type which is able to cause communities concern. This type of marriage has always had its political aspects. States are not very happy about encouraging mixed marriages, particularly if the foreigner maintains links with his own land. They much prefer straightforward naturalisation. The fact is that mixed marriages do not enjoy a status which recognises their existence as such.

The concept of dual nationality which exists in some countries only has a formal legal nature and does not affect everyday life. By this lack of trust from the legal point of view, states reveal the real distances or differences that exist in these marriages. Against the backdrop of various resemblances, be they cultural or social, there are ethnic and particularly religious differences which the partners will have to come to terms with. These differences are sometimes easier to come to terms with in a foreign partner than are cultural and social differences in a partner of the same nationality.

It is above all the religious difference that gives rise to opposition, both from the communities and within the couple itself. Married partners who regularly practise their religion may experience more difficulties than those who only occasionally do so. Indeed religion accounts for many breakdowns in relationships. Areas of incompatibility and ongoing ill-feeling can come to the surface at the slightest provocation, resulting in violent conflicts, and these are sometimes developed into sociolinguistic rifts. There are many examples of this: the old religious wars in France between Protestant and Catholic, and the Crusades. More recently there have been conflicts such as those in the Lebanon, the conflict between the Israelis and the Palestinians, the fighting in Cyprus, and the terrorism in

Ulster: all of these are situations in which religion plays a major role. The people fighting in these battles are separated by their religious affiliation. Indeed religion reinterprets society and justifies actions performed in defence of it, sometimes backed up by overcodified regulations.

It is true that religion has been longer entrenched in some countries than the social classes themselves. More than one hundred and thirty years of colonialism in Algeria did little to alter the deep underlying religious structures.

In many undeveloped countries the socio-religious state of consciousness can be stronger than class consciousness; this is a rare occurrence in industrialised societies.

The first of these groups of countries will condemn marriages between different religions, whereas the second group will not forbid socially mixed marriages, though these will still come up against problems because of the homogamy of the class system.

This type of marriage will therefore raise the problem of the acceptance of its existence in society and that of the decisive influence of the stronger religion for the woman.

Above all, exogamy in a far-off land is only possible for men who have been there in exile for a long time. To acquire women outside of the group is a gain, but to allow a woman to move away is regarded as a loss for the group: a loss of capital and of future enrichment because of her reproductive potential. Indeed, the control exercised over women is aimed at the children she may have; it is she who will determine the continuity of the group: she produces and reproduces the life and traditions of the group. In the relationship between the sexes, the social position of the woman is decisive in determining whether mixed marriages will increase or be reduced in the context of the development of the marriage bond which is geared towards establishing a balance between the minimum of kinship and the maximum amount of emotional investment. A mixed marriage is an example of the institution of marriage in which the differences are more an expression of the differences between the groups than of the differences between the individuals involved.

Partners in mixed marriages in the world today experience a 'mixed condition' which can be quite difficult, depending on where they live. They have to cope with many forms of reserve: from their families, from their friends, from institutions and from the authorities; in some countries they are even forbidden to marry or are subject to strict regulations. Above and beyond recognition of the individuals in their own right, will it ever be the case that the societies and social groups from which the partners in a mixed marriage come will acknowledge the existence of that couple (and their children) in society, in an unconditional way which is not dependent on complete assimilation of the foreign partner? Can mixed marriage only be viable if one of the partners is prepared to conform and to merge with the culture of the country in which the couple lives? It is, of course, recognised that this type of marriage goes against the accepted practice in society. However, social transgression has its positive side. It is often the case that individuals are ahead of institutions. The barriers erected between countries and groups are not always those which separate individuals. It could one day be the case that we will no longer talk of mixed marriages: then it may be the norm to 'marry a foreigner'.

## Marital Distinctiveness

If the institution of marriage is an attempt to safeguard the unity and coherence necessary for reproduction of the society as a whole, mixed marriages also constitute an institution, a whole made up of a number of complementary factors. We should not so much talk of mixed marriage, as mixed marriages.

The 'distinctiveness' necessary at the heart of a couple's relationship is what makes mixed marriage special. It imposes a new structure on the relations between the partners in the framework of a set of practices which leads them to ideas they are both able to accept. As we have seen in the case of language, for example it is the couple's linguistic differences which oblige them quickly to come to an agreement on a minimum common language of communication.

Being aware of the distinguishing characteristics results, not in obstinate hostility and division, but in respect for the other person, in making allowances for the ways in which the other person is different; this positive attitude brings pleasure to the partners as they become aware of the variety in their relationship and enables a husband or wife to say every day: 'He/she never ceases to surprise me'. Far from frantically searching for similarity or accepting a cultivated incompatibility, the distinctiveness we are talking about adds a new dynamic dimension to a couple's relationship.

To be different does not mean to be at loggerheads, nor does it mean being complementary. Disjointed partners? Not any more. Because it is not a question of moving across from an obsession with unity to an obsession with difference experienced in the dull, ongoing linearity of parallel lives.

It is not a question of slavish allegiance to what makes partners different in a marriage. On the contrary, it has to do with replacing the necessarily limited, functional distinctiveness with a qualified distinctiveness which encapsulates the social and cultural aspects of all marriages, in addition to the deep emotional feelings of the two individuals involved.

The partners, who were disjointed at the beginning, progress from the position of being passive partners to the position of being conscious, active partners in areas which are necessarily limited to begin with but which expand with time.

It is precisely this living, coherent combining of the attitudes and practices referred to above, in the context of the various experiences of everyday life, which will bring about the desired dynamics in the marriage relationship.

These partners also know that they are people who have been moulded by their respective social backgrounds, cultures and family structures. They know, in addition, that the dialectic relationship between what and who they are and society in general will in part determine a successful outcome, a stalemate situation or yet again the irredeemable solitude of two people locked into their own worlds.

Marriage is a phenomenon which differs from one society to another, with potential for a distinctive autonomy in each case. We also know that not all individuals and couples have the same opportunities for developing this distinctiveness. It can sometimes be an unattainable luxury. One actually needs certain resources in order to achieve the distinctiveness we have been talking about. It is here that mixed marriage and non-mixed marriage come together. It is individuals — people acting as free agents in society — who are special, not the marriages themselves.

We have come a long way from the idea of marriage for love, in which a chance encounter is blessed with an added measure of happiness . . . On the contrary, this distinctiveness in marriage makes it possible for happiness to become a daily decision.

We live beneath the same roof, but in two different countries.

He has his world, I have mine. There are some things I cannot understand about him, and things he cannot understand about me.

At certain moments we come together on common ground which is not so much a country as a marital no-man's land, a place in which we negotiate our marriage treaties, our many arrangements, assert our rights and conduct quarrels. We try to do this calmly; but even there, in the words themselves, we encounter two different countries.

This is our life. However, this does not prevent us from taking the occasional trip into the other's country. But we never settle there. We quickly retreat to our own territory, where we feel at home.

I can see that in this type of relationship between two people one of the partners is always at an advantage over the other — the one who has been experiencing a deep sense of exile for a number of years. That person will then demand a disproportionate compensation and this demand will not always be met. In this type of marriage there are certain limits and in mixed marriages certain barriers which cannot be passed. It depends to a great extent on what the two partners want, but it also depends on the different mental structures which have been imprinted on their souls.

Though it might not be obvious, there is a certain sense in which it is often the strategies we employ that become this area of minimum consensus.

So our conflicts suffer from the same type of imperfection as our marriage does (French woman, aged 40, married for fifteen years to a foreigner).

# Further reading

The following titles, also published by Multilingual Matters, are of related interest.

Lenore ARNBERG, 1987, *Raising Children Bilingually: The Pre-School Years*.

Hugo BAETENS-BEARDSMORE, 1986, *Bilingualism: The Basic Principles* (2nd edition).

Young Yun KIM, 1988, *Communication and Cross-Cultural Adaptation*.

Gail MELTZER and Elaine GRANDJEAN, 1989, *The Moving Experience: A Practical Guide to Psychological Survival*.

Patricia NOLLER and Mary Ann FITZPATRICK, 1988, *Perspectives on Marital Interaction*.

George SAUNDERS, 1988, *Bilingual Children: From Birth to Teens*.

George SAUNDERS (editor), (quarterly), *The Bilingual Family Newsletter*.

# RAISING CHILDREN BILINGUALLY:
## The Pre-school Years
### Lenore ARNBERG

*"This is a book whose time has come. I welcome it and wish it well and will refer to it often in conjunction with my own bilingual grandchildren . . . I feel indebted to Arnberg, and, I am sure, so will all others who read this book whether they do so for practical or theoretical reasons."* From the Foreword by Professor Joshua Fishman

Covering the many different kinds of family bilingualism that can arise in modern society and written with the needs of parents in mind, this best selling title is essential reading for healthcare personnel, pre-infant school teachers and students of education psychology and linguistics.

*Contents:* Foreword (by Prof. Joshua A. Fishman); 1. Introduction; 2. Immigrant Parents; 3. The Effects of Bilingualism on the Child's Development; 4. Raising Children Bilingually in the Family: Some Research Findings with Regard to the Minority Language; 5. How Children Learn Language; 6. Learning Two Languages: Simultaneous and Successive Bilingualism; 7. Language Strategies in the Family; 8. Family Goals with Regard to Degree of Bilingualism; 9. Practical Suggestions for Raising Children Bilingually Inside the Home; 10. Practical Suggestions for Raising Children Bilingually Outside the Home; 11. Case Studies: Meet Several Bilingual Families.

Paperback 0-905028-70-8    £6.95 (US$15.00)            1987   MM29
Hardback 0-905028-71-6    £20.00 (US$42.00)            168 pages

    **MULTILINGUAL MATTERS LTD**
**Bank House, 8a Hill Road, Clevedon**
**Avon, England, BS21 7HH**   

---

# BILINGUAL CHILDREN: From Birth to Teens
### George SAUNDERS

This sequel to George Saunders' first book, *Bilingual Children: Guidance for the Family* continues the story of bringing up children as successful bilinguals to the age of thirteen. There have been substantial alterations and additions to the original text and a complete new chapter (two varieties of German meet: a family language and a national language) covering the period when the children went to school in Germany for the first time ever. As in the earlier book, introductory chapters cover the theoretical background to bilingualism and these have been modified to include the most recent research material.

This successor to our best selling book ever will certainly receive the same sort of reviews as George Saunders' first book:

"This book represents a remarkable achievement and deserves to be widely known. It goes far beyond a 'how to' book for parents raising their children bilingually. It deserves a wide audience among specialists in childhood bilingualism and among all those generally interested in the psychological, social, and educational consequences of bilingualism."    Glen G. Gilbert in *Language in Society*

"This is one of the most convincing and *most readable* contributions to the field."
*Times Educational Supplement*

Paperback 1-85359-009-6    £7.95 (US$17.00)            1988   MM44
Hardback 1-85359-010-X    £23.00 (US$49.00)            288 pages

    **MULTILINGUAL MATTERS LTD**
**Bank House, 8a Hill Road, Clevedon**
**Avon, England, BS21 7HH**

You may order the books advertised here, or any of our other titles, from your local bookseller.

In case of difficulty, order direct from either of the two addresses below. Please send payment with order for the price of the book(s) or your credit card number and date of expiry if you prefer to pay by American Express, Visa, Access, Euro or Master Card.

Books ordered from the UK should be paid for in Pounds Sterling and from the USA in United States Dollars.

Please add £1.00 (US$2.00) for the first book and £0.50 (US$1.00) for each subsequent book to cover postage & packing.

| MULTILINGUAL | MULTILINGUAL |
|---|---|
| MATTERS LTD | MATTERS LTD |
| Dept B | Dept B |
| Bank House, 8a Hill Road | c/o Taylor & Francis Ltd |
| Clevedon, Avon | 242 Cherry Street |
| England, BS21 7HH | Philadelphia PA 19106-1906 |
| | USA |